The Cleveland Clinic Guide to

BLADDER CANCER

WITHDRAWN

**Derek Raghavan, M.D., Ph.D.,
and Kathleen Tuthill**

Illustrations by Bill Garriott

KAPLAN)

PUBLISH

New Yor

© 2010 Kaplan Publishing

Artwork is reprinted with the permission of The Cleveland Clinic Center for Medical Art & Photograph © 2010.

Published by Kaplan Publishing, a division of Kaplan, Inc.
1 Liberty Plaza, 24th Floor
New York, NY 10006

Library of Congress Cataloging-in-Publication Data
Raghavan, Derek.
  The Cleveland Clinic guide to bladder cancer/Derek Raghavan and Kathleen Tuthill; illustrations by Bill Garriott.
    p. cm.
  Includes bibliographical references and index.
  ISBN 978-1-60714-637-7
  1. Bladder cancer—Popular works. I. Villiers-Tuthill, Kathleen. II. Title.
  III. Title: Guide to bladder cancer.
    RC280.B5R35 2010
    616.99'462–dc22

                                    2009040760

Printed in the United States of America

10 9 8 7 6 5 4 3 2 1

ISBN-13: 978-1-60714-637-7

Kaplan Publishing books are available at special quantity discounts to use for sales promotions, employee premiums, or educational purposes. Please email our Special Sales Department to order or for more information at *kaplanpublishing@kaplan.com,* or write to Kaplan Publishing, 1 Liberty Plaza, 24th Floor, New York, NY 10006.

*To my mother, Betty Raghavan, who faced life
and death with courage and dignity.*

—DR

*To Beth, whose journey inspired me to care about
bladder cancer, and to my parents, who inspired me
to care about writing.*

—KT

And ...

*To all those with bladder cancer and their loved
ones. May you be blessed with hope and excellent
care.*
—Derek Raghavan and Kathleen Tuthill

Contents

Introduction

The bladder is a hollow organ nestled in the lower abdomen that serves as a storage container for urine, the liquid waste produced by the kidneys. The inner tissue of the bladder is surrounded by an outer layer of muscle that tightens to increase the pressure in the bladder when one is about to pass urine, forcing the urine to pass from the bladder into the urethra (the flexible tube that carries urine from the bladder to the point of urination) and out of the body. Cancer that arises in the bladder is one of the most common malignancies in industrialized societies, yet it is not well understood in the community at large. We believe that it is time to provide a simple, nonmedical explanation of this disease for people who have to deal with this illness either as patients or as caregivers.

Cancer can affect any part of the bladder. When bladder cancer is examined under a microscope, different types can be identified. Urothelial cancer (which, for many years, was termed *"transitional cell cancer"* or *TCC*), which accounts for more than 90 percent of bladder cancers, begins in the innermost layer of bladder tissue and consists of cells of variable sizes and shapes. It has been called "transitional" because it resembles some of the other patterns of cells that are found in other bladder cancers and has been thought to be intermediate or transitional between some of them. Because of where it begins, i.e., the lining of the bladder or "urothelium," it is now more commonly called *urothelial cancer.* Another pattern is *squamous cell carcinoma,* which starts in the flat cells that line the inside of the bladder and (under the microscope) closely resembles the appearance of the cells that make up the layers of skin. *Adenocarcinoma* begins in cells that have a glandlike appearance and make mucus. Squamous cell carcinoma and adenocarcinoma are very uncommon.

Cancer is not one disease; it is many diseases affecting parts of the human body. All cancers have one thing in common: something has gone wrong in the way some of the body's cells normally grow, divide, and die. When a cancer forms, the main problem is that some cells start to grow, slowly or quickly, in an uncontrolled fashion, and the usual switch-off mechanisms that stop cell growth don't work properly. The breakdown in the switch-off mechanisms may be caused by exposure to chemicals (e.g., some of those found in cigarette smoke), radiation, or even rare types of virus infection. The extra cells may cluster and form a tumor. Cancer cells may invade and damage surrounding tissue. Cancer cells may also break away and spread through the body by entering the lymph or blood systems. Most bladder cancers that are located on the inner surface of the bladder are treated by techniques that kill them or remove them surgically. Bladder cancers that are invasive (having burrowed into the wall of the bladder) or metastatic (having spread to other parts of the body) require more complicated treatment, as the following chapters will describe.

Bladder cancer primarily affects people between the ages of 50 and 75, and more often men than women, and more Caucasians than African Americans, Hispanics, or Asians. Smokers, former smokers, and people whose jobs expose them to certain chemicals or environmental toxins are at higher risk of developing bladder cancer. Family members of people who have had bladder cancer are at *slightly* higher risk of developing the disease, and if you have already had bladder cancer, you have an increased chance of getting it again.

In this book we'll look at all aspects of bladder cancer and what you can expect at each step of the treatment process. We'll talk about symptoms, tests, diagnoses, treatments, recurrence probabilities, clinical trials, drug treatments, support groups, questions you'll want to ask your doctor, and how to interact with hospitals, insurance companies... and yes, even doctors.

Most important, we'll help you understand bladder cancer and how it might affect your life or that of a loved one, and we'll explore the resources available to you as you continue your journey.

Derek Raghavan, M.D., Ph.D.
Kathleen Tuthill

Chapter 1

The Bladder

T he bladder is a balloon-shaped, muscular organ tucked into the pelvis and held in place by fibrous bands and muscle. The bladder is part of a system that includes the kidneys, ureters, and urethra. These organs process the waste products left behind after your body has taken out the nutrients it needs from the food you eat.

The bladder is lined on the inside by a tissue known as *urothelium,* the smooth layer that stretches as the bladder fills and prevents excreted material from being reabsorbed into the body. Underneath the urothelium is a mix of fibrous or supporting tissue and muscle, both of which help the bladder to expand (when full) and to contract and excrete urine at the appropriate time.

In addition to lining the bladder, urothelial tissue also lines other parts of the urinary tract system, including in the ureters (the tubes that drain the kidneys), the urethra (the tube that drains urine from the bladder to the exterior of the body), and parts of the male prostate. Urothelial tissue can sometimes develop cancerous changes known as *urothelial malignancy*. The most common type of cancer of the urothelial tract is *transitional cell carcinoma, also known as urothelial cancer* (see chapter 3).

When urothelial tissue is exposed to cancer-causing substances, such as the by-products of cigarette smoke, the potential exists for cancerous changes to occur in multiple locations. That's why when bladder cancer is suspected or confirmed, the entire urinary tract is screened for the possible presence of other cancerous deposits.

Other organs, such as the lungs, liver, skin, and intestinal tract, also process waste. These systems work together to balance the chemicals and water your body needs to function properly.

The urinary system processes urea, a specific waste product that is produced when protein-containing foods (such as a meat) are broken down in the digestive process.

Urea is filtered through the kidneys and, together with other waste by-products and water, is converted into urine. Urine is carried by thin tubes called *ureters* to the bladder, where it is stored. Muscles in the walls of the ureters squeeze out small amounts of urine into the bladder on a constant basis, about every ten seconds. A healthy bladder can hold about two cups of urine for up to five hours. Healthy adults produce about six cups of urine a day.

A strong muscle somewhat like a rubber band encircles your bladder and keeps the urethra tightly closed until nerves in the bladder signal you that the bladder is full and it is time to urinate. Urinary problems include the inability to retain the urine in the normal fashion or to void urine from the body. Sometimes people experience the urge to urinate even if the bladder is not full. Sometimes this is caused by bacteria in the bladder, which can cause an infection called *cystitis*. This symptom can also be caused by local bladder irritation or by the development of cancer. Sometimes it is not even related to the bladder but an enlarged prostate, due to benign or cancerous causes. As with all parts of the human body, the bladder can develop cancer, which can also cause problems with retaining or voiding urine.

Symptoms

The most common symptom of bladder cancer is *hematuria,* or blood visible in the urine, either with or without any accompanying pain. About 80 percent of the people diagnosed with bladder cancer notice blood in their urine, and it's often what prompts them to seek medical attention.

In some cases, the presence of blood isn't noticeable to the naked eye and can only be seen through a microscope, usually when a urine test is being done during a routine physical or when an infection of the urinary tract or bladder is suspected. A urine test can detect whether blood is present in the urine and can also rule out whether other things, such as food or medicines, are the cause of red or rusty-colored urine.

Noticeable blood in the urine is a tricky symptom. It can appear in varying colors and at irregular intervals, and as a result, you might overlook its significance or decide to wait and see whether it happens again before seeking medical attention.

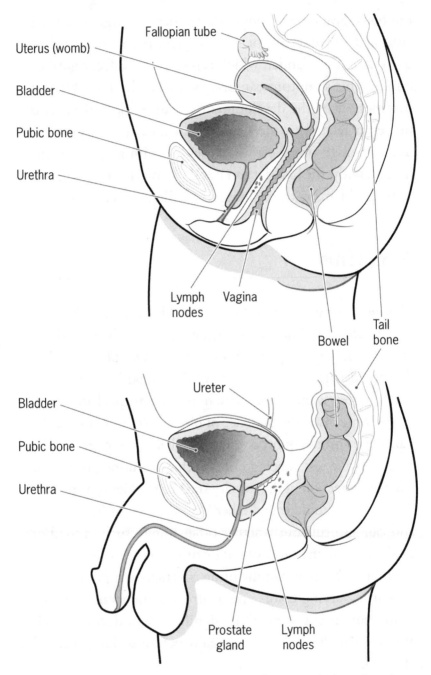

Figure 1.1— *Side views of the bladder and surrounding organs in the male and female anatomies*

For example, you may notice blood in your urine or drops of blood in your underwear two or three times in as many days, or you may see it on one occasion but after that your urine appears normal for days or weeks. The same thing can happen during a laboratory urinalysis, where red blood cells may be visible microscopically only intermittently.

You might experience a gush of bright red blood or notice pink or rusty brown urine or even little clots of blood. To complicate things, foods such as beets or blackberries may produce colored urine, as do a number of medicines, food additives, and vitamins.

With the major symptoms of bladder cancer acting in such a variable fashion, appearing in different ways and sometimes disappearing altogether, it's important to see your doctor immediately if you notice blood or what you think might be blood in your urine. As with most cancers, the key to successfully managing bladder cancer is detecting it early and starting treatment as soon as possible.

Bladder cancer does not produce many symptoms, and many of the symptoms are typical of other, less severe conditions, such as infections or benign tumors. Besides blood in the urine, your symptoms can include pain or burning during urination, a feeling of having to urinate because of an uncomfortable fullness, or the need to get up frequently at night to urinate.

You may also have symptoms such as backache, abdominal pain, and unplanned weight loss, or you may feel more tired and achy than usual.

Who Gets Bladder Cancer?

The most significant factors that put you at high risk of developing bladder cancer are age, sex, history of exposure to cigarette smoke, and occupation. The American Cancer Society estimates that in 2009, about 70,980 new cases of bladder cancer will be diagnosed in the United States (52,810 men and 18,170 women).

Men are at much higher risk for bladder cancer than women, although it's not known why; it strikes men three to four times as often as it does women. The American Cancer Society projects that men have a 1 in 27 chance of developing bladder cancer, while women have a 1 in 84 chance. The good news is that overall death rates for bladder cancer are decreasing for both men and women.

Bladder cancer is the fourth most common cancer among men in the United States (following prostate, lung, and colon cancers). It is most common in people between the ages of 50 and 75, and is rarely diagnosed in children.

Caucasians constitute the group at highest risk for developing this form of cancer, followed by African Americans. For reasons that are not yet known, fewer Asians develop bladder cancer. U.S. government statistics show that about 40.3 per 100,000 Caucasian men and 9.9 per 100,000 Caucasian women will be diagnosed with bladder cancer compared to 20.0 African American men and 7.9 African American women.

Schistosomiasis, a parasite common in some Middle Eastern countries (particularly Egypt), is linked to a type of bladder cancer known as *squamous cell carcinoma*. The parasite isn't picked up by casual visitors, but instead may affect those who have traveled there for long periods or lived in the Middle East for any length of time. This latter group is at higher risk for schistosomiasis and its subsequent chronic irritation of the bladder, which can eventually result in tumors.

Most significant in the list of risk factors is exposure to cigarette smoke. It is estimated that up to 80 percent of all bladder cancers can be attributed to cigarette smoking, your own or possibly even someone else's, if you were nearby to inhale it ("passive smoking" or "secondhand smoke").

Bladder Cancer by the Numbers

Statistics compiled by the U.S. government between 2004 and 2006 show that 2.41 percent of the men and women born today will be diagnosed with urinary bladder cancer.

Between 2002 and 2006, Incidence Rates per 100,000 Population

	Men	Women
All Races	37.1	9.3
White	40.3	9.9
Black	20.0	7.9
Asian/Pacific	16.5	4.0
American Indian/Native Alaskan	12.4	3.4
Hispanic	19.8	5.3

(continued on next page)

Between 2002 and 2006, Mortality Rates per 100,000 Population

	Men	Women		Men	Women
All Races	7.5	2.2			
White	7.9	2.2	American Indian/		
Black	5.5	2.8	Native Alaskan	2.7	1.1
Asian/Pacific	2.7	1.0	Hispanic	3.9	1.3

Probability of Developing Bladder Cancer between Ages 50 and 70 Based on 2004–2006 Statistics

Men	1.19 percent	Women	0.34 percent

If you were raised by smokers or live in a house with smokers, you may be at risk, as are people who are current or former smokers. To a lesser extent, smoking pipes or cigars also carries a risk. Snuff and chewing tobacco have not been linked to bladder cancer.

The risk of bladder cancer quickly drops when you quit smoking. However, as a former smoker you remain at risk because it can take 20 or 30 years for bladder cancer to manifest itself. Certain variables, such as how deeply you inhaled cigarette smoke and how long you smoked, can elevate or reduce your risk.

Occupational exposure to certain chemicals accounts for up to 20 percent of bladder cancers. Some of those chemicals, such as the benzidine used in the textile dye and rubber-tire industries, have been banned in the workplace. Other suspected *carcinogens* (cancer-causing substances), such as 4-nitrobiphenyl, 2-naphthylamine, and 4-aminobiphenyl, are no longer produced in the United States; however, previous use in some occupations may have put workers at a higher risk for bladder cancer. Those occupations include:

- Laborers in textile dye, rubber, and chemical industries with exposure to aromatic amines
- Some pharmaceutical or pesticide manufacturers
- Workers employed in coal or gas production
- Painters
- Truck drivers
- Hairdressers
- Sewage workers
- Metalworkers in the aluminum, iron, and steel industries

Other risk factors include chronic urinary tract infections, exposure to cyclophosphamide or ifosfamide (chemotherapy drugs used for certain cancers), and pelvic radiation for cervical cancer. There is also a somewhat elevated chance of developing bladder cancer if a member of your family has had the disease. Although there is evidence that saccharin consumption is a risk factor, various studies have failed to find a strong link between bladder cancer and caffeine or modern artificial sweeteners. People who consume lots of fluids have been reported to have a lower incidence of bladder cancer, perhaps because fluids flush cancer-causing chemicals out of the bladder.

The most recent cancer research indicates that bladder cancer might be prevented through changes in lifestyle, so don't use tobacco products and be sure to limit your exposure to certain chemicals, drugs, and radiation.

Some risk factors, such as heredity, can't be controlled, but you can be aware of them and of any symptoms of diseases that have appeared in previous generations of your family. Keep in mind that even if an inheritable disease is present in your family history, it doesn't mean that everyone in your family will actually *get* the disease. In fact, most won't. But because you have an increased *likelihood* of developing the disease, you can and should get regular checkups so if cancer does develop, you'll catch it early, at a stage when treatment is most effective.

Max

Max worried when his urine was a rusty brown color one morning, but he put off doing anything about it at first. He still worked part-time at Maple Grove's water-treatment plant, and the U.S. Environmental Protection Agency was due any day to make its annual inspection. He needed to be there, keeping tabs on his crews and making sure that there were no glitches when the EPA team arrived.

Besides, everything was fine the next time Max went to the bathroom. Normal. Yellow. It didn't hurt when he urinated, although it did burn a little sometimes and he found himself getting up four or five times a night to go to the bathroom. He attributed the change to getting older.

When the rusty brown urine appeared again a few days later, he told his wife, Jean, who immediately called the doctor's office. The nurse told Max to take a urine sample to the lab the next morning and made an office appointment for two days after that.

At the Urologist's Office

When Max came in to see Dr. J, the nurse asked him a number of questions. When did the symptoms start? How would he describe the color of the urine? Were any clots of blood visible? Any pain when he urinated? Had he ever had blood in his urine before? Did he feel any itching or burning? Any fever?

She performed the usual blood-pressure check, declaring it "perfect," and left his file, complete with her notes from the questions she asked Max, tucked into the holder on the front of the examining-room door.

Blood in his urine? Max immediately jumped to the conclusion that the nurse had seen the results of the urine test and knew it was blood. Max had suspected as much but hearing it out loud . . . well, that was scary.

When Dr. J entered the examination room, he asked the same questions the nurse had, plus a few more. Was Max getting up frequently at night to urinate? Did his bladder feel full, even when he didn't have to urinate? Had he had any unplanned weight loss? A cough?

Max, who was feeling very anxious by now about what might be wrong with him, lashed out at Dr. J.

"You know, I just answered these questions for your nurse. Doesn't anyone here write things down? Or read what does get written down?"

Dr. J smiled. "Max, doctors are trained to get information right from the source—the patient—even if there are detailed notes made by a nurse or another doctor. It's easy to make a wrong assumption or to misinterpret someone else's information, and that could adversely affect my diagnosis or treatment plan for you. I guess from your point of view, it seems as if we don't communicate. But really, we're just trying to get it right."

Max nodded. "Okay. I can understand that. It just seems sometimes that the same things are asked over and over, and it gets frustrating." Feeling calmer, he asked, "What else do you want to know, Doc?"

"How about smoking? You quit a few years ago, didn't you?" Max admitted that he still smoked a few cigarettes a day, although not in his house. His wife wouldn't let him.

"Good for her. Smoking or living with a cigarette smoker puts you and her at risk for all kinds of health problems. I want you to get serious about quitting, Max. Very serious."

Dr. J performed a physical exam and then told Max to get dressed and come down his office to talk. Max didn't like the sound of that.

Urinalysis: Three Categories

Routine urinalysis examines the urine. It falls into three categories: macroscopic, dipstick, and microscopic.

Macroscopic Urinalysis Macroscopic urinalysis is visual observation of the color and clarity (or cloudiness) of the urine.

(continued)

Dipsticks Dipsticks are plastic or paper strips coated with chemicals that change color if certain substances (such as glucose, protein, or blood) are present in the urine. Dipsticks provide immediate results and are cost-effective, but they provide limited information. For example, a dipstick test can confirm the presence of protein in the urine, but it doesn't measure the quantity. More accurate measurements can be made on collected urine by a chemical analyzer, a machine that can measure the presence of sugar, protein, or other substances in the urine.

Microscopic Urinalysis For detailed analysis of the cells present in urine, a microscopic urinalysis is performed. For this test, urine is prepared in a laboratory—usually by being spun in a centrifuge to separate out the various cells (which are heavier than water or urine, and sink to the bottom of the tube), which can then be examined under a microscope for the presence of blood cells, cancer cells, or bacteria.

To prepare for a urinalysis, you should avoid heavy athletic activity or physical labor the day before the test, since extreme activity can sometimes result in the appearance of small amounts of blood in the urine. Collect the urine first thing in the morning, if possible, in a sterile, covered container. (This is usually provided by the doctor's office or laboratory.) Thoroughly wash the area around the urethra (the body opening where urine exits the body). Let the first few drops of urine fall into the toilet; this clears the urethra of any remaining contaminants. Catch a few ounces of urine in the clean container, and if you are not able to give it immediately to a nurse or laboratory assistant, store the urine in a cool place. (Your refrigerator is fine.) Make sure you get the urine sample to the doctor's office or laboratory within four hours.

In some cases, your doctor may want to use a catheter (a thin, flexible tube) to take a urine specimen directly from

(continued on next page)

the bladder. This procedure can be done in your doctor's office with a minimum of discomfort. Your doctor will use a local anesthetic cream to numb the tip of the penis and, in both men and women, the urethra.

Some medications discolor or cause false results in a urinalysis. Make sure your doctor has a list of all medications you take regularly, including over-the-counter antacids or pain relievers, vitamins, calcium and other minerals, and herbal supplements or teas.

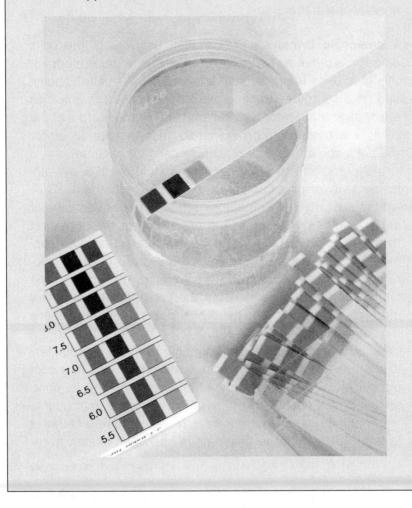

Dr. J usually spoke to Max right there in the examining room. Max threw on his clothes and hurried down the hall.

"Max, I want you to see a urologist at the Glickman Urological and Kidney Institute at Cleveland Clinic. The results of the urine test show some red blood cells in your urine, and given what you've told me today about your symptoms and history, I think further tests are in order to rule out certain conditions. I'm more comfortable having a urologist do those tests."

"So what do you think the problem is?" Max asked. "Something with my kidneys?"

"I think more likely it's bladder disease, Max."

"Like an infection or something?"

"That's possible, but I don't think it's very likely. We need to rule out a few things. This could be a benign condition, such as an infection, or it could be bladder cancer. I know that's a scary thing to hear, but there are lots of red flags that put you in a high-risk category, including your age, sex, occupation, and symptoms, and the fact that you are a smoker. If it is bladder cancer, Max—and right now we don't know that it is—the sooner we treat it, the better."

Dr. J explained the tests the urologist would want to do and gave Max a pamphlet about bladder cancer and how it's diagnosed.

"I know it's easier said than done, but don't start worrying yet, Max. The urologist will eliminate the possible causes of the red blood cells in your urine, and we'll go from there. Let's see what the tests show."

For a brief moment, Max wished that Jean hadn't called Dr. J. Then he wouldn't have heard the words "bladder cancer" and wouldn't be feeling sick to his stomach. What would having cancer be like? Would he have to have surgery? Chemotherapy?

Max took a deep breath. "Okay, I guess I'd better go see the urologist."

The urologist scheduled an ultrasound and intravenous pyelography (IVP). He told Max that depending on the results, he might schedule more tests. (Note to the reader—the details of all these tests and what they entail are described in chapter 2.)

Max underwent the IVP test first. He grumbled about having to fast in the morning and grumbled even more about the effects of the laxative he had to take the night before the exam.

The test itself, he admitted, was a breeze. Other than a prick from the needle for the IV and a nasty metallic taste in his mouth while the X-rays were being taken, the IVP procedure was, according to Max, "a piece of cake."

For the ultrasound, Max had had to drink a large amount of liquid so his bladder would be full during the test; this made it easier to get a good reading. The test itself wasn't painful or unpleasant.

It took two weeks for the series of tests to be completed and the results delivered to the doctor. Max spent many sleepless nights worrying. Most of the time he could be optimistic about his future, even if he was diagnosed with cancer. But in the middle of the night, when Jean was sleeping and the house was quiet, Max got scared, deep down, gut-level scared. *What if it is cancer? What if I'm going to die?*

Finally, the time came for Max and Jean to return to the urologist's office to receive the test results. The urologist told them that Max did, indeed, have bladder cancer, but that the tumor was limited to the surface of the bladder (he called it "superficial") and noninvasive.

Max let out a sigh of relief. He had convinced himself that the news would be more serious.

The doctor explained that Max's tumor was confined to the urothelial (transitional cell) epithelium. Treatment, he said, would consist of a small surgical procedure (a "resection") to remove the tumor, followed by a series of bladder washes made through a urinary catheter, using an immunological treatment called Bacille Calmette-Guérin, or BCG, to help make sure the cancer didn't recur. Max turned to Jean and said, "Well, it looks as if you're stuck with me another few years."

"I can deal with that," said Jean, tears trickling down her cheeks. The doctor cautioned Max and Jean that the word *superficial* wasn't interchangeable with *harmless*.

"Superficial urothelial cancer is highly treatable, but it has a high recurrence rate, Max. Sometimes it recurs at a more serious level. I don't want to alarm you, as there is every reason to expect a good outcome in your case, but I do want you to be aware of the possibility of recurrence and to impress upon you the importance of follow-up."

The urologist continued, "If your cancer does come back, it's likely to happen during the first two years after surgery, so we're going to keep a close eye on you, Max. We'll do urine tests and flexible cystoscopies regularly. And I want to know right away if you have any symptoms such as blood in your urine or painful urination, or if you're more tired than usual or have any new aches or pains, or a persistent cough."

Max was still floating on the hopefulness of his diagnosis. It was Jean who answered. "Don't worry, I'll keep him honest."

Smoking-Cessation Resources

- The **American Cancer Society** sponsors the Great American Smokeout each November and posts resources about quitting smoking at www.cancer.org. You can also call the American Cancer Society's national number 800-227-2345 (800-ACS-2345) for information, or check your phone book for your local American Cancer Society office.

- **The American Heart Association** makes available books, tapes, and videos about quitting smoking. Information can be found at www.americanheart.org or by calling 800-242-8721. You can also check your phone book for information about your local American Heart Association office.

- **The American Lung Association** offers a self-help quit program called Freedom from Smoking. Find information about Freedom from Smoking at www.lungusa.org or by calling 800-586-4872 (800- LUNG-USA). For information on local American Lung Association offices, check your phone book.

- **Ask your doctor** about the advisability of using over-the-counter or prescription nicotine patches, gums, and other products as part of your program to stop smoking. Also ask for information about local groups that sponsor smoking-cessation programs or support groups.

- **Cleveland Clinic** has been very active in promoting smoking cessation and has been completely smoke-free since July 4, 2005. In addition, it provides smoking-cessation programs and assistance for patients and staff. Information is available at myclevelandclinic.org/tabacco/default.aspx

(continued)

- **The National Cancer Institute** website—www.cancer.gov—provides a link to information about quitting (www.smoke-free.gov). It also has a telephone quitline (877-448-7848). Live help with questions about or problems associated with quitting smoking is available at the NCI website by clicking on the LiveHelp link at www.cancer.gov.

Chapter 2

Diagnosis and Tests

A fter taking a patient's history and performing a physical examination, among the first steps most physicians take to diagnose bladder cancer are a urinalysis and some or all of the following tests: intravenous pyelography (IVP), an ultrasound, and X-rays, followed by a flexible cystoscopy. These tests are described later in this chapter.

Typically the IVP and ultrasound are the first steps in the diagnostic process. However, in some circumstances, doctors prefer to perform the flexible cystoscopy first.

Sometimes your family doctor will schedule these tests (although a urologist will perform a cystoscopy, if it's needed); sometimes your doctor will refer you to a urologist for all the tests. It's not important from your standpoint whether the urologist or a family doctor does the tests, so long as the tests are completed.

Urologists at Cleveland Clinic

Most family doctors or internists will refer you to a urologist at some point in the initial diagnostic process. At Cleveland Clinic's Glickman Urological and Kidney Institute, the urologists are highly trained specialists who are experienced in the treatment of urinary tract disease, including bladder cancer. Usually board-certified and licensed in the urology field, these doctors are up-to-date in the latest diagnostic and treatment methods. The Glickman Urological and Kidney Institute is ranked No. 2 in the United States and has been a top urological center for many years.

It's important to note that the diagnostic progression does not unfold in exactly the same order for all patients. Which tests are ordered and when they are performed will depend to some degree on the results of each previous test. Besides the tests mentioned above, some or all of the following procedures may also be used in the diagnostic process: a CAT or CT scan, an MRI scan, an inpatient or outpatient cystoscopy, and surgical biopsy. (Each of these procedures will be discussed in this chapter.)

What to Expect during the Initial Diagnostic Process

If you scheduled an appointment with your doctor because of any of the symptoms described in chapter 1, your doctor will take a detailed history, perform a full physical examination, and probably schedule a urinalysis and perhaps additional tests.

During your office visit, your doctor will ask you detailed questions about your lifestyle, symptoms, and medical history. Your doctor may ask you questions that don't seem relevant to your symptoms, such as whether you are experiencing abdominal pain or your bones ache more than usual, and whether you've unexpectedly lost weight or developed a cough. The doctor is looking for indications that cancer might be present elsewhere in the body; such indications will determine which tests he or she will recommend.

Routine body functions such as lung, heart, and blood pressure should be checked. Your abdomen should be examined, and for men, a prostate exam should be performed, while women should expect a vaginal exam.

At this point, the doctor may schedule further tests or refer you to a urologist.

The descriptions of procedures and test processes or preparations that follow are of a general nature; your experience during your actual process, preparation, or procedure may differ from what is described here.

Flexible Cystoscopy

When you are referred to a urologist, he or she will review your history and perform a careful physical examination. The urologist may then suggest a *flexible cystoscopy.* This procedure allows the urologist to look around inside your bladder for the presence of small tumors or abnormalities without doing an invasive, or surgical, procedure. Flexible cystoscopy is usually performed in your physician's office under local anesthetic, although in some cases, the urologist may prefer to conduct a similar procedure, called a rigid cystoscopy, which involves using a larger, more rigid device, under general anesthesia in a hospital setting.

Cancer has the potential to arise at any part of the urothelial tract (the lining of the bladder, ureters, and urethra), so the urologist will carefully examine the whole of the bladder and will sometimes use a different scope—one with a smaller gauge—called a ureteroscope to examine the upper urinary tracts (ureters). This procedure is simply an extension of the cystoscopy, using a slightly different gadget, and is not painful.

If your doctor scheduled an IVP first and tumors were observed, the flexible cystoscopy test may be omitted and other tests may be recommended for you as the next step in the diagnostic process.

During the flexible cystoscopy, a thin, flexible tube with a lighted lens or fiber optic is inserted into your bladder through the urethra. To minimize pain, a local anesthetic in the form of a cream or gel is gently applied in the urethra first. A sterile liquid, usually a saline solution, flows through the cystoscope, filling and stretching your bladder. You may feel some fullness and the urge to urinate during a cystoscopy. It helps alleviate discomfort if you relax your abdominal and pelvic muscles.

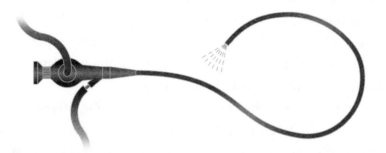

Figure 3— *A flexible cystoscope*

During a cystoscopy, your doctor watches the images transmitted from the bladder by the cystoscope. The images appear either through a lens or on a computer screen. Sometimes urine that is in your bladder at the time of cystoscopy will be collected for examination, or a tissue sample may be taken for biopsy.

Your doctor will also digitally examine your bladder with a gloved finger, from the rectum if you are a man and also from the vagina if you are a woman, to determine whether there is any thickening of your bladder wall, which can be an indication of an invasive tumor. Pressing gently with the finger, the doctor can feel abnormalities in the wall or position of the bladder.

Patients sometimes describe feeling some abdominal pressure or discomfort, but not pain, during the flexible cystoscopy procedure. You will be awake, wearing a gown and lying on an examining table, with your knees draped and positioned apart. As noted above, your doctor will use anesthetic gel to numb the area where the flexible tube is

inserted and then gently guide the cystoscope into the ure-
thral opening (the eye of the penis in a man; the vaginal
outlet of the urethra in a woman). Some men experience
brief pressure and discomfort as the cystoscope passes over
the area where the prostate is located.

In most cases, the entire process, including preparation,
will take about 15 to 20 minutes, and your doctor will be
able to discuss the results of the flexible cystoscopy with you
immediately.

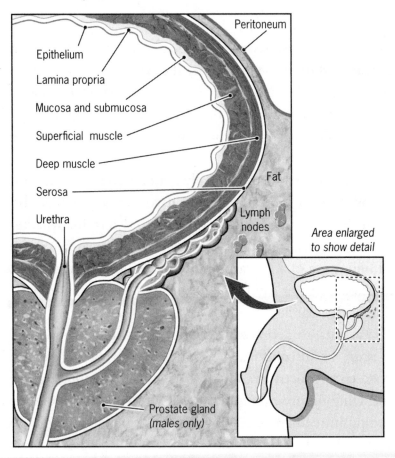

Figure 4—*The layers of the bladder wall*

Rigid Cystoscopy

A rigid cystoscopy may be performed when a tumor is located in an inaccessible part of the bladder as well as when a more complicated biopsy is needed. It is performed in a hospital setting as either an inpatient or an outpatient procedure. The process is similar to flexible cystoscopy, but you will be given general anesthesia and a more rigid tube will be used.

Your doctor will give you specific instructions about how to prepare for the anesthesia (you will need to have someone drive you to and from the hospital) and what to expect during the brief recuperation after the procedure. You may be asked to remain overnight if you have other medical problems, such as severe heart disease.

Intravenous Pyelography (IVP)

Intravenous pyelography is a form of X-ray. It is painless except for the pinprick from the intravenous needle. The IVP test and all of the following X-ray or scan procedures are performed by a radiologist and radiology technologists at your hospital's radiology department or at a recommended imaging center.

The IVP helps physicians see most cysts, stones, abnormalities, or tumors in the bladder. Because small tumors don't show up on an IVP but may be visible during a flexible cystoscopy, both procedures may be used as diagnostic tools.

During the IVP, you'll be lying on a flat table, wearing a hospital gown, with the X-ray machine positioned above you on a movable jointed arm.

The radiologist will take some basic X-rays and then will inject a contrast substance (usually iodine) through a vein, usually in your arm. The iodine is carried by the blood system to the kidneys, where it is removed (excreted into the urine). The iodine shows up when exposed in an X-ray. Be sure to notify the doctor in advance if you know that you are allergic to iodine or if you have had an allergic reaction to some type of X-ray procedure in the past.

You might feel a sense of heat or burning from the iodine or have a metallic taste in your mouth. However, these sensations usually disappear after a few minutes. If you know that you are allergic to iodine, let the radiologist know and a different contrast material can be used.

As the iodine travels through your urinary tract a quick series of X-rays is snapped. Sometimes the radiologist will apply a gentle compression elastic band around your body to help the visualization process. You may be asked to turn over and might even be asked to empty your bladder. (The iodine should not cause any discoloration of your urine or any pain or burning during urination.)

The X-rays taken before the iodine was injected and those taken after provide images for your doctor that give a visual picture of the ureters (the tubes between the kidneys and bladder) and the bladder's anatomy and function.

Ultrasound

Your doctor may also recommend an ultrasound, sometimes called a sonogram, to help examine your bladder.

An ultrasound, as its name suggests, is an imaging process that uses high-frequency sound waves that bounce off organs such as the bladder to create a visible image. It's a painless, very safe procedure that usually takes less than a half hour to complete.

You'll be lying down on an examining table, wearing a gown and covered by a drape. A technologist will smear a clear gel over your abdomen. The gel often feels clammy and cold, but it's necessary to help transmit the sound waves.

The technologist then moves a transducer (an imaging gadget shaped somewhat like an oversized electric shaver with a flat head) over the area where the bladder is located. You probably will be asked to change positions or even to hold your breath for a few seconds during the process. The technologist watches on a screen to make sure that clear images are being recorded.

The Next Step in the Diagnostic Process

If any test suggests the presence of a bladder tumor, your doctor will schedule other tests, which might include an MRI or a CT scan, and if a biopsy was not obtained during the flexible cystoscopy process, a surgical biopsy as well. These tests help your doctor determine where the tumor is, what type of cancer you have, and whether the cancer has invaded the muscle wall of the bladder. Depending on the results of those tests, your doctor may order a chest X-ray or even a bone scan to determine whether the cancer has spread to other areas of the body.

Computed Tomography (CT or CAT Scan)

A CT scan is a painless, noninvasive test during which low-intensity X-rays are repeatedly passed through the body's soft tissue at different angles. A computer then processes the X-rays to show a detailed cross section of the tissues and organs—in your case, of the bladder, liver, spleen, abdominal lymph nodes, and surrounding tissues. Sometimes the scanner will be focused on the chest and lungs to see whether cancer has spread there.

From the CT scan, your doctor usually can confirm the presence of a tumor in the bladder, and can measure its size and location and determine whether it has spread to other, nearby tissue.

The CT scanner is a large rectangular machine with an opening for an X-ray "tube" that will move around your body, snapping images that the computer will assemble into a set of cross-section scans that can be viewed by the physician. These scans show remarkably clear images of the various organs. The scanner usually makes a whirring sound as it moves and a click similar to a camera as it snaps images.

The CT scanner can snap about 32 cross-section pictures or "slices" in approximately ten seconds as the machine moves over your body. This means that you can easily hold your breath as the images are taken.

For the CT scan, you'll be lying on a table, dressed in a gown, and while you'll be able to talk with the radiology technicians at all times over an intercom, you'll be alone in the room and asked to lie still and hold your breath while the actual X-rays are being taken.

Like the IVP, a contrast medium is used to help the radiologist see your bladder and urinary tract. Sometimes the medium is injected into the veins, as in IVP, or it may be swallowed or sometimes administered as an enema to distinguish bowel tissue from the bladder structure. Usually when diagnosing bladder cancer, doctors will want all three—intravenous, oral, and rectal scans—to determine how deeply tumors may have invaded the bladder tissue and whether there is any spread to the abdominal lymph nodes or liver.

Some people find the taste of the contrast medium unpleasant, and if an enema is required, you are likely to feel a brief, uncomfortable fullness while the scans are being taken. However, because of the speed of the process, the feeling that you need to expel the contrast medium doesn't last long. You might also feel a brief flush or hot sensation when the contrast medium is injected.

A CT scan takes anywhere from 5 to 30 minutes. Other than mild discomfort, there are few side effects.

Nuclear Magnetic Resonance Imaging (NMR or MRI) Scan

Sometimes doctors request an MRI instead of a CT scan. Like the CT scan, an MRI is painless and noninvasive, but

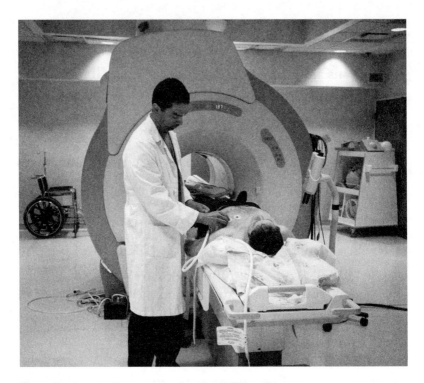

Figure 5—*A magnetic resonance imaging (MRI) machine*

unlike the CT scan, no radiation is involved. An MRI uses radiofrequency waves and an electromagnetic field to stimulate atomic nuclei in the body. The energy released by these nuclei is recorded and provides an accurate visualization of soft tissue in your body.

The MRI machine is a big metal box with a tunnel through its middle and a narrow sliding table. You'll lie on the sliding table, which will move you slowly through the electromagnetic field or tunnel of the MRI machine. An MRI can take anywhere from 15 to 45 minutes. Some MRI machines are closed cylinders; others have wider tunnels and open sides to reduce the claustrophobic feelings that some people experience. If you suffer from claustrophobia—the fear of close or enclosed spaces—you should warn your doctor that you might not be comfortable having an MRI scan.

You'll wear a gown, and as with the CT scan, the radiology technicians leave the room during the scanning process, but you'll be able to communicate with them through an intercom. Sometimes a friend or relative is permitted to sit in the room with you, particularly if you are claustrophobic. If you are claustrophobic, your doctor may give you a gentle sedative to help you to feel comfortable in the machine.

Sometimes a contrast medium is used, usually intravenous, in which case you might experience a cool sensation. You'll be asked to remain very still for short periods while the images are being taken, usually anywhere from a few seconds to a few minutes at a time. You'll be able to move slightly between takes or images.

Other than what many patients describe as a closed-in feeling, the single most uncomfortable part of an MRI is not being able to move about. Patients also comment that MRIs can be surprisingly noisy. Sometimes you'll also hear a banging sound as the scans are being taken. Many physicians feel that MRI scans are a useful alternative to CT scans, but results can be more difficult to interpret when the MRI scan is focused on the back of the abdomen, the pelvis, and bladder, so generally CT scans are more frequently used.

Surgical Biopsy

Usually performed under general anesthesia in a hospital, a biopsy via a rigid cystoscope allows the physician to examine your bladder manually for any abnormalities (again, by inserting a finger into the rectum and feeling the local tissues) and then to remove small amounts of tissue. The tissue samples can be examined microscopically to confirm the presence of cancer and the invasiveness of the disease, as well as to help determine the appropriate treatment.

Sometimes, in the case of small or superficial tumors, the physician will remove the entire tumor and surrounding tissue for biopsy. As with all surgeries or invasive procedures, a biopsy may involve some pain as well as a brief recovery time that might call for some limitations on physical activities for a day or two. The urologist will prescribe pain-relieving medication to reduce discomfort.

Other Tests

If your test results suggest that the cancer may have spread to other organs or areas of the body, your doctor may schedule a chest X-ray or bone scan.

Getting a Second Opinion

You may want to seek a second opinion about your diagnosis. In fact, some insurance companies require you to get a second opinion, even though you might be worried about delaying your treatment. Don't be. A brief delay while you gather your records and talk to another doctor or medical team shouldn't be a problem.

(continued)

How do you go about finding another doctor for a second opinion?

- First, you might ask your doctor for a recommendation to another expert who can give a second opinion.
- You can call the National Cancer Institute at 800-422-6237 (800-4-CANCER) for information about treatment centers the organization supports.
- You can check with your local medical society, a nearby hospital, or even a medical college if one is nearby. Most states have National Cancer Institute –designated Comprehensive Cancer Centers, and doctors at such institutions will usually provide a second opinion.
- The American Board of Medical Specialists has a publication—*The Official ABMS Directory of Board Certified Medical Specialists*—that lists certified doctors. The list is also available online at www.abms.org. (Click on "Is Your Doctor Certified?")
- Two annual publications, *America's Top Doctors* (published by Castle Connolly; www.castleconnolly.com/books/index.cfm) and *Best 100 Doctors in America,* both list prominent cancer specialists whose peers have identified them as experts. The *Best 100 Doctors* list is compiled by bestdoctors.com, launched in 1989 by doctors affiliated with Harvard University. The list is not released to the general public. Instead, the list is provided to designated regional magazines and to hospitals. Check with the health center where you plan to receive treatment to find out which of its doctors may be included on this list.

A **chest X-ray** is a type of X-ray process that takes about ten minutes. You'll wear a gown and remain standing during the X-ray. The radiology technician will ask you to stand in several positions and will take X-rays of the chest area.

It's a painless process and doesn't require that you drink or be injected with any contrast medium. This test can indicate whether the cancer has spread to the lungs and also can reveal other, unrelated medical conditions, such as a chest infection.

A **bone scan** requires a very small amount of a radioactive tracer, which is injected into the bloodstream. Bone absorbs the tracer, which gives off gamma rays; these are then scanned to identify areas of abnormality. The purpose of this test is to monitor for the presence of cancer metastases in the bones, but it can also detect infection or arthritis.

A bone scan is a time-consuming test. It takes about three hours for bone to absorb the tracer after it's injected into your vein (usually in an arm). After the tracer is injected, you'll leave for a few hours or wait in the waiting room (bring a book). The scan itself takes about an hour.

During the scan, you'll lie on a stationary table while a big cylinder—actually a gamma camera—moves up and down the table as it takes pictures. The cylinder doesn't enclose you to the extent that a MRI machine does and usually doesn't provoke a claustrophobic feeling. As with a CT or MRI scan, you'll lie on a table, wearing a gown, and will have to remain still when the gamma camera is clicking away, sometimes for several minutes at a time. You'll be asked to change positions several times during the scan, usually a welcome relief after you've had to remain motionless.

Sometimes tests of the urine are done to determine the presence of biomarkers. These are proteins that may be released by bladder-cancer cells into the urine. One example is the **NMP22** or **BladderCheck** test. For this, a few drops of voided urine are tested chemically on a glass slide. Some physicians believe that the NMP22 is more sensitive and more accurate than the more conventional cytology test, in which urine is examined for cancer cells under a microscope.

After the Tests Have Been Completed

Once all the test results are available, they will be carefully evaluated by your doctor and the radiologist. In addition, your doctor may suggest adding an oncologist to your medical team at this point.

The next step will be for you and your family to discuss with the doctor the results of the tests and the biopsy, and to determine the course of treatment that is right for you.

If you had symptoms that suggest possible bladder cancer, make sure your physician checks you out thoroughly. If, for example, IVP results don't show the presence of any tumors, it may be wise to get a second opinion if the symptoms persist without any explanation. If all tests are negative, generally no further follow-up is necessary unless your symptoms—particularly the painless passing of blood in the urine—occur again.

Tests, Risks, and Precautions

Following are some additional details about the tests your doctor may order.

Flexible Cystoscopy

This 30-minute test is performed in the doctor's office. You'll return home without assistance the same day. Discomfort is minimal.

Preparation: A local anesthetic, usually a gel, is applied before the procedure. You'll wear a hospital gown.

Risks: The test is generally safe. There is possibility of infection or bleeding; rarely, there is perforation of the bladder.

After-effects: You should drink plenty of fluids. You may experience burning during urination and a small amount of blood may be visible. If either continues after 24 hours (or if blood continues to appear after voiding has occurred three or more times), your doctor should be informed. If you are unable to urinate, the doctor should be contacted or you should go to a hospital emergency department.

Precautions: An allergic reaction to the sterile fluid or anesthetic gel is possible. If you are taking a blood thinner, you must inform your doctor.

Rigid Cystoscopy

This surgical procedure is performed in the hospital while you are under general anesthesia (i.e., asleep). Recovery time is brief; if you are able to urinate, you will go home the same day. (You'll need a driver.) You will need to rest for 24 hours and your activity will be restricted for a short time. Mild discomfort may limit some activities.

Preparation: Fasting is necessary, usually for a minimum of 12 hours prior to surgery. Antibiotics may be prescribed.

Risks: The procedure is generally safe. There is possibility of infection, difficulty urinating, bleeding, swelling, or (rarely) perforation. Occasionally, urinary retention occurs, requiring a catheter. Complications from anesthesia are possible.

After-effects: Pain is minimal. Swelling or burning may occur during urination. (These reactions are normal.) Blood may appear in the urine, occasionally for as long as three weeks. You should call your doctor immediately (or go to an emergency department if he is not available) if fever or excessive bleeding occurs, clots appear in the urine, testicular pain develops, or urination is not possible.

Precautions: If you are taking a blood thinner (e.g. Coumadin or warfarin), you must inform your doctor *before* the procedure.

Intravenous Pyelography (IVP)

This outpatient procedure is performed at an imaging center or hospital radiology center. It can take as long as 60 minutes (possibly longer). It is noninvasive and discomfort is minimal.

Preparation: The test is preceded by a 12-hour fast. A laxative may be prescribed for the evening before the test. You'll wear a hospital gown. All jewelry or metal must be removed.

Risks: An allergic reaction to the contrast medium or iodine is possible. There is a very low risk of exposure to radiation.

After-effects: You may experience a mild itching, or hives may appear. If the condition persists, you should notify your doctor.

Precautions: If you are pregnant or nursing, inform your doctor. Tell your doctor about any allergies (especially to shellfish) that you may have. If you are diabetic, let your doctor know. And tell your doctor about any medications you are taking.

Ultrasound

This test is performed at an imaging center or hospital radiology center. It usually lasts less than 30 minutes. It is non-invasive, and any discomfort is very minimal.

Preparation: You'll have to fast for several hours before the test. Usually, you wear a hospital gown. An hour before the test, you must drink and retain four to six glasses of fluid.

Risks: There is a very low risk of allergic reaction to the conducting gel.

After-effects: There are no after-effects.

Precautions: If you have any allergies or have recently undergone a barium X-ray, your doctor should be informed.

Computed Tomography (CT or CAT Scan)

This test is performed on an outpatient basis at an imaging center or hospital radiology center. It usually takes

60 minutes or less, but it may last up to two hours. It is noninvasive and there is minimal discomfort. If you require a sedative, you will need to arrange to be driven home.

Preparation: Preparations can vary. A fast of up to 12 hours is usually called for. For some scans, you must take a laxative or enema the night before. You may need to have a blood test of kidney function in advance. You may be asked to drink a contrast solution before the test. You'll wear comfortable, loose clothing (without zippers or snaps) or perhaps a hospital gown. All metal objects (such as jewelry, hairpins, dentures, and hearing aids) must be removed.

Risks: The test involves very low exposure to radiation. An allergic reaction (rarely serious) to the contrast material used in the test is possible.

After-effects: During the test, you may feel warm or flushed, have a metallic taste in your mouth, or experience a headache or slight feeling of nausea. For 24 hours after the test, you should drink plenty of fluids.

Precautions: If there is any possibility that you may be pregnant, the doctor should be told. If you are nursing, you should discuss with your doctor the precautions to take with breast milk and ask for added advice about precautions with the baby. The doctor should be told if you have allergies (especially to iodine); are asthmatic; have problems with your kidneys, heart, or thyroid; have multiple myeloma; or take metformin for diabetes.

Magnetic Resonance Imaging or Nuclear Magnetic Resonance Imaging (MRI)

This test is performed at an imaging center or hospital radiology center. It usually takes as long as 60 minutes but may last as long as two hours. It is noninvasive. (However, an intravenous line may be used.) Discomfort is minimal, beyond the occasional discomfort at being confined. If you are claustrophobic, you should notify your doctors; you may require sedation or an open body-scan machine. If you are going to receive a sedative, you should arrange for a driver to take you home after the test.

Preparation: You may wear comfortable, loose clothing (without zippers or snaps) or perhaps a hospital gown. All metal objects (such as jewelry, hairpins, dentures, and hearing aids) must be removed. Some people bring earplugs or headphones to use during the test.

Risks: An undetected metal implant may react to the strong magnetic field. There is a low risk of allergic reaction to the contrast fluid used in the test.

After-effects: If you have metal fillings in your teeth, you may feel a tingling in your mouth. Reactions during the test may include slight nausea, vomiting, headache, dizziness, pain, burning, or breathing problems.

Precautions: Let your doctor know if you have a prosthetic limb or hip; a pacemaker; an IUD; an artificial valve; an implanted port catheter; or any metal pins, plates, screws, or surgical staples in your body. Tell your doctor about any allergies or medical conditions you may have. If you are (or may be) pregnant or wear a medication patch, tell your doctor. If you are claustrophobic, let the doctor know when you schedule the test. Also tell your doctor if you have any tattoos.

Surgical Biopsy

This is performed in association with cystoscopy. It can be done on an outpatient basis or as an overnight stay.

Preparation: Patients usually need to fast for several hours before the procedure, so check with your urologist when you schedule the test. Jewelry should be left at home.

Risks: The procedure is generally safe. You may have some lower abdominal pain postbiopsy and may note blood in your urine for a few days.

After-effects: You may feel some burning during urination as well as postbiopsy discomfort or pain. Analgesics should be used as prescribed.

Precautions: The doctor should be told of persistent bleeding or pain or other unexpected symptoms. On rare occasions, an inability to pass urine may require a temporary urinary catheter.

Chest X-Ray

This test is performed at an imaging center or hospital radiology center. It usually takes about ten minutes.

Preparation: You wear a hospital gown and must remove jewelry or metallic objects from the waist to the neck.

Risks: There is a low risk of radiation exposure.

After-effects: There are no after-effects.

Precautions: If you are nursing or there is any possibility of pregnancy, the doctor should be told in advance.

Bone Scan

This test is performed at an imaging center or hospital radiology center. The test itself usually takes about an hour; however, waiting time for the absorption of the tracer and between scans can be as long as six hours (sometimes you will receive the injection of scanning material and be allowed to go home for a couple of hours, rather than just waiting in the radiology center).

Preparation: In most cases, no X-ray studies using barium should be performed in the four days leading up to a bone scan, as barium may interfere with the quality of the bone scan images. Fluid intake should be limited for four hours before the test. A hospital gown is worn, and jewelry and metal objects must be removed.

Risks: There is a low level of exposure to radiation. Reactions may include rash or swelling. Severe allergic reaction (anaphylaxis) is possible.

After-effects: If occasional soreness or swelling occurs at the injection site, apply warm, moist compresses. If a rash develops or the swelling worsens, tell your doctor.

Precautions: If you are nursing or there is any possibility of pregnancy, tell your doctor in advance. The doctor should also be told about any allergies.

What to Ask Your Doctor about Tests

These are by no means all the questions that may occur to you, but they will get you off to a good start.

What is the name of the test I am having?
Why do I need this test?

Your doctor's answer should include the full name of the test and whether the test is to diagnose disease or confirm a diagnosis, to help determine a course of treatment, or to eliminate certain medical possibilities or the possibility of other diseases.

Will I need other tests? Will you repeat this test?
How urgent is it that I have this test now?

Your doctor's answer should explain whether the results of this test may indicate that more tests will be needed, what those tests are, and why this test might need to be repeated. During the diagnostic process, the doctor will consider it important, if not urgent, to have you undergo tests that will help confirm your condition and plan a treatment.

What do I need to do to prepare for the test? What side effects or risks might there be? How long is the test likely to take?

The descriptions in this chapter are only a guide, and your doctor may offer more detailed instructions or require a different selection of preparatory steps. Answers should, in general, be similar to the precautions and preparations outlined in this chapter.

How much does the test cost? Is it covered by insurance?

Your doctor may refer you to his office staff for information on cost and insurance coverage.

Where will the test be done, and what certifications are held by the facility doing the test?

The office staff may schedule the test for you and give you directions to the radiology center, if needed. The imaging center should be certified by the American Board of Radiology, which ensures that its staff is properly trained to handle equipment that is inspected and certified as safe. When you are discussing qualifications of doctors or technicians, listen for the words *board-certified* or *certified by the board,* along with references to the American Medical Association, American College of Surgeons, or American Board of Radiology.

When will you get the results?
How will you communicate the results to me?

Your doctor will estimate how long it will take to get the test results. Your doctor is likely to suggest scheduling an appointment for you and your family to come in and discuss the results and their implications for you and your treatment plan. That's the ideal way to review the results. However, if you are more comfortable talking on the phone, then you might want to request a phone call instead.

Be cautious about asking questions if you aren't likely to understand the meaning of the answer. For example, if you ask, "Where did you do your residency?" the answer probably won't mean much to you unless you have some idea of which hospitals or universities provide high-quality training.

The key is to ask the questions that are important to you. If you want to know how you'll feel after a test, that's the question to ask. If you want to know whether you should eat a special diet or change your work habits, ask that.

What to Tell Your Doctor

When your doctor is considering a diagnosis of bladder cancer, what you do for a living and how you spend your time are important pieces of information. If your physician doesn't know where you've worked or what your job history is, make sure you talk about this information, because these facts may give him or her a clue about what caused you to develop bladder cancer.

If you have never mentioned that you started smoking again after quitting 15 years ago, now is the time to confess. It is clear that once bladder cancer has been diagnosed, continuing to smoke is an adverse outcome factor (in other words, the results of treatment are worse for people who continue to smoke).

If you have worries about little aches and pains, speak up. That occasional ache in the lower left abdomen might be an important signal to your doctor, even though you are convinced that it only happens when you carry the garbage

(continued on next page)

cans out to the curb on Tuesdays. If you experience a little burning when you urinate or notice a brownish discoloration sometimes, tell your doctor.

Think about things that may have changed in your habits or your life. Do you have to take a nap every day, when just a year ago you were full of energy? Do you drink more water now? Or consume three alcoholic drinks instead of one? Are your feet always cold? Do you take a herbal remedy, such as feverfew or black cohosh? Do you have much more indigestion or heartburn than you used to? Have you been losing weight?

You don't need to bombard your doctor with every detail of your life, but do mention your family history, changes in how you feel, what hurts, and any new symptoms you are having.

Chapter 3

What the Tests Tell Your Doctor

When the Test Results Arrive

You have undergone a battery of tests. A flexible cystoscopy. An IVP, a CT scan, perhaps even a surgical biopsy and bone scan. The diagnosis? You have bladder cancer.

Although you may well have reason to be hopeful about your treatment and outlook, the words are serious and frightening. Most people diagnosed for the first time with bladder cancer have tumors that are limited to the bladder itself. In about 20 percent of first-time cases, the cancer will have spread deeply into the bladder wall or to surrounding tissue outside the bladder, and in roughly 3 percent of the first-time diagnoses, it will have spread to other organs and tissues in the body.

Bladder cancer isn't just one disease, however, and what type of cancer you have, how deeply it's embedded in the layers of the bladder, and whether it is superficial or invasive and has spread to other parts of the body are all important pieces of information to you and your doctor, not only to predict the progression of the disease, but also to determine what treatment is right for you.

Different types of cancer respond differently to different types of treatment, so it's important for your medical team to evaluate your test results carefully before deciding on a treatment plan.

What are doctors looking for when they evaluate your test results? They are looking for the *type* of cancer you have, the *appearance* and *shape* of the cancer cells, whether the cancer is *superficial* (also termed *noninvasive*) or *invasive,* the *stage* of the cancer (how invasive into the bladder wall the cancer is), the *grade* of the cancer (how abnormal the cancer cells appear under the microscope), and whether *multiple* types of tumors are present.

Types of Bladder Cancer

Bladder tumors are grouped into several types, according to the way the tumors appear under the microscope. Three common types of bladder cancer are:

- **Urothelial cancer,** or UC (also referred to as *transitional cell cancer* or *TCC).* It can be localized on the surface or it may be invasive. (UC will be discussed in more detail later in this chapter.) UC is the most common type of bladder cancer, accounting for about 90 percent of all cases. In 2009, the American Cancer Society estimated that by the end of that year about 70,980 people would be diagnosed with bladder cancer—roughly 52,810 men and 18,170 women. About 63,882 of the cases would be urothelial cancer.

- **Squamous cell cancer.** This type of cancer accounts for about 4 percent of all bladder cancers and is usually an invasive cancer. *Squamous* means "resembling a scale" (which is flat and thin) or a scaly surface, and squamous cell cancer looks like skin cancer when viewed under a microscope. Among the causes of squamous cell development is the *schistosomiasis* parasite discussed in chapter 1.

- **Adenocarcinoma.** The appearance of this type of cancer closely resembles tumors of gland-forming cells in the intestinal tract. (*Adeno* means "gland.") It is often associated with the production of small amounts of mucus. Some adenocarcinomas occur in the urachus, a remnant of a fetal structure that connects the bladder to the umbilicus before birth. Adenocarcinomas, which are usually invasive, account for about 1 to 2 percent of bladder cancers.

In addition to the above types of bladder cancer, there are several extremely uncommon forms of the disease:

- **Small cell anaplastic** bladder cancer. Similar to small cell cancer, this rapidly growing cancer is usually found in the lung, and it shares a pattern of rapid growth and early spread to other parts of the body. It is not really clear why small cell tumors arise in the bladder, although it is thought that they start from neuro-endocrine cells, isolated small, dark, round cells that arise during fetal development, of uncertain function, which are sometimes found in the bladder. These cells may play a part in the control of cellular growth.

- **Sarcomas** and **choriocarcinoma**. It is quite rare for these two forms of cancer to be found in the bladder. Sarcomas are found in the muscle layers of the bladder. Choriocarcinoma is most often diagnosed among Asians in the Far East. Found in the bladder wall, it is an extremely rare tumor that seems to arise from small clusters of cells that paradoxically resemble part of the placenta.

Squamous cell, adenocarcinoma, and other rare forms of cancer are generally diagnosed and treated in much the same way as muscle-invasive bladder cancers, and their treatment will be discussed in chapter 5.

Urothelial Cancer (UC)

A diagnosis of urothelial cancer (also known as transitional cell cancer) can mean many different things. Urothelial cancer is not a single type of cancer; it is classified by shape and whether it is restricted to the inner surface of the bladder (superficial to underlying tissues and muscle) or invasive, as well as by stage and grade of development.

The words *transitional cells* describe how the cells appear under the microscope. Transitional cells share features with various types of cells normally found near the bladder. Since 2009, pathologists have altered the common term to "urothelial cancer" to acknowledge the fact that all these cells arise from the lining of the ureters, bladder, and urethra, the urothelium.

The human bladder is composed of several layers. On the innermost surface (which is next to where urine is stored) is a layer of cells known as the *transitional cell epithelium.* This layer varies in thickness from three to seven cells.

If your doctor described your tumor as being confined to the transitional cell epithelium, the tumor is a superficial tumor. About 74 percent of UCs are noninvasive and superficial when diagnosed, although superficial tumors may eventually progress to a more invasive stage. The word *superficial* has to be used carefully because it does not necessarily mean that the tumor is safe and doesn't have a dangerous potential. In other words, some "superficial" tumors actually have a high malignant potential and the ability to spread elsewhere in the body.

A diagnosis of invasive UC means that the cancer has progressed into other layers of the bladder wall, such as the intermediate cell layer or the muscle.

Shapes of Bladder Cancer

Urothelial cancer is classified as either papillary or flat in shape, although and more than one kind of tumor may be present at the same time in the bladder.

Papillary tumors look like the fronds of a fern or a bunch of tiny berries or grapes. Papillary tumors can be superficial or invasive. Most papillary tumors are malignant; however, the papilloma tumor is a relatively benign type of papillary UC and is typically removed by surgery.

Other tumors appear to be flat and velvety and are more commonly called carcinoma in situ (CIS). These tumors are only one cell thick.

Staging and Grading of Bladder Cancer

When you met with your doctor to discuss your diagnosis, he or she probably described your cancer stage with a combination of letters and numerals, which you may not have understood.

Staging is a way to determine how deeply your cancer has penetrated into the bladder and muscle, surrounding tissue, or distant organs. The pathologist stages the tissue

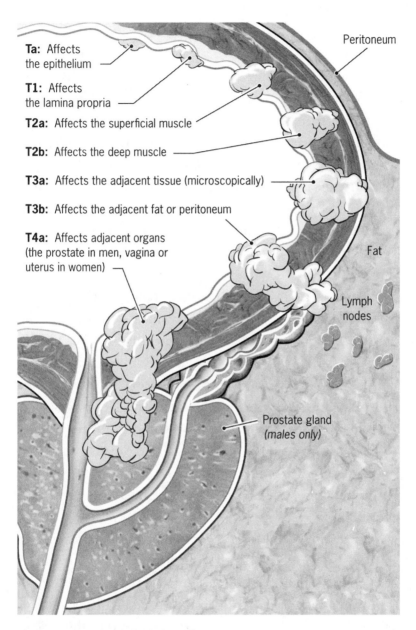

Ta: Affects the epithelium

T1: Affects the lamina propria

T2a: Affects the superficial muscle

T2b: Affects the deep muscle

T3a: Affects the adjacent tissue (microscopically)

T3b: Affects the adjacent fat or peritoneum

T4a: Affects adjacent organs (the prostate in men, vagina or uterus in women)

Peritoneum

Fat

Lymph nodes

Prostate gland (*males only*)

Figure 6—*The stages of bladder cancer as it progressively invades the layers of the bladder wall and surrounding organs*

from your biopsy, and your doctor uses that information along with your scan, cystoscopy, and X-ray results to determine where you are in the disease process and what treatment is best for you.

If the results of your tests—either scans or biopsies—show that cancer has spread to other tissue or organs, your doctor will want to confirm that. Clarification of the stage of your cancer comes through looking at the cancer cells from those organs under the microscope. Tissue samples may be taken at the time of your biopsy, or sometimes a needle biopsy is done, bypassing the need for additional surgery.

Pathologists stage bladder-cancer tissue by using a standardized system known as TNM, which stands for *tumor-nodes-metastases*. A typical TNM might be "T2aN1M0" (T-two-a-N-one-M-zero). Looks like mumbo jumbo, doesn't it? Try thinking of it as medical shorthand, with each letter and numeral having a defined value that gives doctors and pathologists a specific, consistent way to describe how deeply a cancer has invaded the body's tissue and organs.

The TNM system uses the letters *T, N,* and *M* followed by numerals to describe the stage of invasiveness of your cancer.

The letter *T* followed by a numeral from one to four (1 to 4) describes the depth of invasiveness of your tumor. The lower the number, the less invasive the cancer.

The T scale has additional, more detailed levels as well. These levels add the lowercase letters *a* and *b* to the T score to delineate more precisely how far into the bladder your cancer has spread and whether it has moved into other areas of your body. It fine-tunes the pathology information to help your doctor make treatment recommendations.

The first T level refers to Ta or T1 tumors, which are superficial in nature. These noninvasive tumors can be papillary or carcinoma in situ (CIS), and have penetrated only the epithelium or intermediate cell layers of the bladder. This is an early, highly treatable stage of bladder cancer. The Ta tumor is the least invasive (or most superficial) variant, whereas the T1 tumor shows the beginnings of invasion into the first layer of the bladder wall (before muscle is reached).

Tumors that are invasive and have moved into the muscle layer of the bladder are classified as T2. The lowercase letters *a* and *b* are used to describe how far into the muscle the tumor has spread. A T2a tumor has not penetrated as deeply into the muscle as a T2b tumor.

Tumors classified as T3, which can be further classified by the letters *a* and *b*, have penetrated beyond the bladder wall and into the fatty tissue surrounding the outside of the bladder. A T3a tumor is visible only with a microscope. A T3b tumor is visible in scans or to the naked eye during surgery.

A T4 tumor, the most serious and advanced of this local tumor grouping, has spread to other tissues or organs. A T4a tumor has invaded the nearby uterus or vagina in a woman or the prostate in a man. A T4b tumor has spread through the pelvic or abdominal wall into the body.

The letter *N*, followed by a numeral from one to three (1 to 3), tells your doctor whether your cancer has spread to lymph nodes near the bladder and how deeply the cancer has penetrated the nodes. The higher the number, the more lymph nodes are involved and the more enlarged the nodes are.

The letter *M* followed by a one or a zero (1 or 0) indicates whether your cancer has spread to lymph nodes in other parts of the body (beyond the pelvis) or to other organs such as the lungs or liver. A zero indicates that the cancer has not spread to other organs; the number one means that it has.

Once your doctor and pathologist have determined your TNM values, the results will be combined and expressed as Roman numerals from zero to four (0 to IV). Stage IV, for example, is the most advanced and serious stage of cancer. The stages help predict rates of survival five years after treatment; they range from 98 percent survival in the Stage 0 category to about 15 percent in the Stage IV category. The stage of your cancer also helps doctors decide how aggressive to be in recommending treatment options.

The terms *Stage I* or *Stage IV* are like medical shorthand, giving your physician a quick indication of overall prognosis and the general type of treatment that will be needed.

Grading tumors is another tool for your doctor. Instead of measuring how invasive the tumor is, grading indicates how abnormal the tumor cells appear under the microscope. The more abnormal, or undifferentiated, the tumor cells are, the more likely it is your cancer will spread aggressively.

Pathologists use the numerals one, two, or three (1, 2, or 3) or the words *low, medium,* or *high* to describe how abnormal the tumor cells appear. A tumor graded three (3) or higher is the most likely to spread aggressively. In some systems, grading is done on a scale of one to four.

Some tumors, including carcinoma in situ (CIS) tumors, are considered a high-grade bladder cancer because they characteristically have a high rate of progression to muscle-invasive tumors and also because they don't have any differentiated features. The paradox is that they are only one cell thick, which usually correlates with *lack* of invasion. About 50 percent of the people diagnosed with CIS who have no other types of tumor present in the bladder will eventually have the CIS invade the muscle.

Recently, an extensive body of research work has suggested that abnormalities (known as "mutations") of the genes that control the growth of bladder cancer may be important in helping to determine the prognosis of bladder cancer. While this is not yet routinely applied to clinical practice, preliminary studies have suggested that mutation of such genes as the P53 gene may be associated with more aggressive behavior of the tumor, with a greater tendency to spread. The P53 gene, which is part of the genetic makeup of the tumor, normally acts to suppress tumor growth; in some cancers, when an abnormality or mutation occurs, that tumor suppressive role is lost.

Other genes may also be involved in this process, including those known as the Rb gene, P16 gene, and a gene that controls the epidermal growth factor receptor (EGFR). As this book is being written, a major clinical trial is studying whether these preliminary observations are true, and the final results are not known. We mention this to encourage you to discuss with your own physician the current state of the art of measuring genes and comparing the results with the outcomes of treatment of bladder cancer.

What Does All This Mean to You?

Physicians and researchers can draw some general conclusions about bladder cancer and its diagnosis and treatment, but it is not always easy to predict how it will behave in a given individual.

Your physician and oncologist work with the pathologist to get an idea of your likely prognosis that is as accurate as possible, but the reality is that tumors of the same type don't always develop or progress in the same way. Nor do vthey always respond to treatment in the same way, and they don't always follow a predictable pattern of recurrence.

Generally, one can say that the more deeply into the bladder layers cancer has spread, the more likely it is to recur. But some superficial cancers become invasive. And some don't. Doctors and researchers don't yet have all the key indicators to predict which superficial cancers will become invasive and recur and which ones won't.

In general, if you have been diagnosed with superficial urothelial cancer, you can expect a 40 percent chance that the cancer won't recur, especially if you have a low-grade tumor where the cancer cells closely resemble normal bladder cells.

Caring4Cancer

Talk with your doctor about whether the publication Caring-4Cancer, a magazine chock-full of information and articles of interest to cancer patients, their families, and caregivers, is right for you. Free copies of the publication are available in bulk only to doctors or health-care professionals at www.Caring4Cancer.com.

- **The Cancer Survivors Network** is a forum or message board at the American Cancer Society website (www.cancer.org) where people can ask questions and share information and resources with other people who are dealing with cancer.
- **Your hospital's social work department** will have counseling and resources available for you and your family. Just ask your doctor to put you in touch with the appropriate office.

Talking with Your Family about Cancer

You'll need to talk to the members of your family about your diagnosis and treatment plans. Here are some pointers to keep in mind:

- Let your family, especially children or grandchildren, know what's happening. Children, even very young children, pick up on worry and anxiety, and easily imagine the worst if information is kept secret.

- To the extent that you are comfortable doing so, share your feelings, and encourage your loved ones to share theirs.

- Take advantage of available resources. There are excellent websites and books available about coping with cancer. (See the section on resources at the back of this book for an extensive list.) You can also ask your doctor to refer you to a social worker or support group.

- When possible, couch discussions in hopeful and reassuring words by telling your loved ones that you feel positive about your treatment.

- When talking about cancer with children, keep information age-appropriate. The National Cancer Institute offers a guide called *Tips for Talking with Children of Different Ages,* which you can obtain at www.cancer.gov.

- With your family members, agree to give each other permission to feel stressed or worried or angry—or even happy—without feeling guilty.

- Acknowledge that there may be tough times ahead, but recognize that caring and love will help get you through them.

- Acknowledge that things will change. Talk about changes as they occur.

- Talk often with family and loved ones. Speak from your heart.

- Expect lots of questions. Expect some disagreements. Expect times when you wish that things could go back to the way they were before you had cancer. And expect deeply meaningful moments with the people you love most.

Diane

Diane knew something was wrong when her family doctor left a message on her voice mail to call about her test results. Usually after her annual physical she'd receive a letter that said "Everything's fine, see you next year."

By the time she got through to Dr. W, her stomach was churning with worry.

"Diane, your urinalysis showed some microscopic amounts of blood in your urine. It's something I think we should check out. Have you noticed any visible blood in your urine or had any changes in urine function? Do you feel that you have to go more often? Do you feel any pain when you urinate?"

Only the previous day Diane's husband had complained that she couldn't shop for more than ten minutes without heading for a bathroom. But she wasn't experiencing any pain or noticing visible blood. That was good, wasn't it?

Dr. W agreed that it was a good sign but still felt Diane should see a urologist.

"It may be nothing more than bladder irritation from the analgesic you take for your arthritis, Diane. But because of your increased urge to urinate, I want to err on the side of caution. Let me switch you to the appointment desk."

At the Urologist's Office

Diane didn't expect Dr. H, the urologist, to do much more than talk during her first visit. So she was surprised when the doctor, after asking Diane a number of questions, including whether she ever smoked and what she did for a living, said that she wanted to perform a flexible cystoscopy. Even though the doctor explained the procedure and assured her that she'd feel fine afterward, Diane was glad that her husband, Carl, had driven her to her appointment.

The flexible cystoscopy wasn't as unpleasant as it sounded, although Diane was uncomfortable when the doctor filled her bladder with fluid and asked her to hold it in.

A few minutes into the procedure, the urologist said, "I'm going to snip some tissue, Diane. You shouldn't feel anything except some minor discomfort. There is an abnormal growth in the upper right quadrant that I think we should biopsy."

After the cystoscopy, which was over in less than ten minutes, Diane hurried to the bathroom to void the liquid she'd been holding for what seemed like hours. Then she met Carl in the doctor's office. Diane mentioned that there had been a little blood in her urine, but Dr. H assured her that that was normal after a biopsy and explained what Diane and her husband should expect next.

"As I told you, Diane, there is tissue with an abnormal appearance in your bladder, which means that there is a significant probability that the growth is cancer. However, we won't know for sure until we get the biopsy results. That will take about a week. In the meantime, I'd like you to have a few more tests so we have a thorough picture of what's going on with you."

Even though Diane had been expecting bad news ever since the doctor had told her during the cystoscopy that there was a growth present, the word *cancer* hit her like a sucker punch.

"Are you sure it's cancer?" Diane asked.

"As sure as I can be without seeing the actual biopsy results, Diane. What I'm not sure about right now is what stage the cancer is or whether it may have spread. That's what these other tests, along with the biopsy, will help us determine."

Both Carl and Diane were stunned. Diane had been feeling fine, and until some lab tech had found a few drops of blood in her urine a week ago, she thought her health was great. Now, in the space of a few days, she was learning she may have cancer. It was hard to process.

Carl said, "Is bladder cancer … a bad kind of cancer? I mean, some types are pretty treatable."

"It really depends on the biopsy results, Carl. There are different types of bladder cancer, some very treatable and some very aggressive. Sometimes we catch it very early, yet the outcome is not what we'd like. We just don't have enough information yet to know in Diane's case."

The urologist asked questions about Diane's weight and energy level. Was she having any new or persistent aches and pains?

Diane replied that she was fine, no problems, but Carl reminded her that she had complained recently about a pain in her abdomen.

Diane could tell that Carl's comment concerned the doctor.

"What are you thinking? That maybe the cancer has spread?" Diane was afraid of the answer, but she asked anyway.

"I don't know what it means right now, Diane. It could be nothing more than gas in your abdomen. Let's get the tests going and take a look at the results before we start jumping to conclusions." Dr. H tapped her pen on the folder and said, "I'm going to write orders for a chest X-ray, some more blood work, and a CT scan."

After explaining the test procedures, she gave Diane brochures about bladder cancer.

"I know this is all overwhelming right now," she said. "I encourage you to think about what we've discussed today. Read the brochures I gave you and make a list of questions. When we've got all the information from the tests, we'll sit down and go over it all together in detail. I'm going to have my staff make your test appointments before you leave and schedule another appointment with me a week after your last test."

"That long? I'll go crazy," said Diane. "Can't we hurry it up?"

"It's hard to wait, I know, but I need time to get the reports back and look them over. In the meantime, try not to worry. Keep in mind that you're 56 and that overall your health is good. These are very positive things working in your favor."

Dr. H stood up and said, "Call my office any time you have questions. I can't always stop and talk to you right then, but I'm very good about returning phone calls. If you're worried about something, even if it's something minor, I want to know. Okay?"

Within minutes, all the appointments were scheduled and Diane was handed preprinted sheets with instructions on what to eat and what to avoid before the tests.

During the ride home, Diane felt as if she were looking at different scenery in a different world. On one hand, everything seemed the same, but sharper. Crisper. The air was cold and fresh, the sky more blue than it had been on the ride to the urologist's office. Yet she also felt focused inward, slightly removed from everything that was happening around her. It took an effort to speak, to listen to and understand what she was hearing, as if all her energy were being pulled into a fragile center from which the word *cancer, cancer, cancer* was drumming through her head. Even though Carl was sitting right beside her, Diane felt very alone.

Over the next two weeks, Diane joked to Carl that she was taking her clothes off and putting them back on so many times that she was tempted just to wear her bathrobe to future appointments. The only test that bothered her was the CT scan; she reacted to the contrast solution the technician injected into her vein and itched like crazy for the next few days, but the reaction subsided quickly after she contacted the doctor, who gave her a prescription for an antihistamine.

With each test, Diane became more worried. If I could just forget about all this for a few hours and get some sleep, she thought, it would be easier. Carl wanted to tell their daughters what was happening, but Diane flatly refused.

"Carl, it's hard enough to keep myself from flying to pieces over this, and you … well, sometimes you look at me as if I'm about to dissolve in front of your eyes. The girls have their families to take care of, and they'd be so upset. Just wait until we know what we're facing. Please? I don't want to worry them any more than is necessary."

Carl agreed, but she still caught him looking at her with a sad, frightened look. She realized that whatever the diagnosis turned out to be, it wouldn't be just *her* diagnosis. It would be Carl's and their daughters', too.

Telling the Family

Diane and Carl sat down to an early dinner with their three adult daughters and their husbands. Diane still felt shell-shocked about the test and biopsy results. She and Carl had decided to tell all three girls about what was happening at the same time, when they were all together. The girls knew something was up, though. It was unheard-of for Diane to invite the adults to dinner without the grandchildren.

After dinner, Carl poured coffee for everyone. Diane took a deep breath and said, "Dad and I have something to tell you."

Despite her best intentions, Diane started to cry. Carl took over. "Mom has been diagnosed with bladder cancer," he said, holding Diane's hand. "It's a kind of cancer called 'invasive cancer,' and it's not a good kind of cancer to have. It's what the doctors call 'high grade,' and it's pretty advanced."

"How advanced?" asked Neil, a pharmacist. "It's Stage III," Diane said. Then, with a weak grin, she added, "You probably want the details. It's a T3aN1M0 tumor."

Neil nodded, and Carl went on. "But … the doc thinks there's a good chance that surgery and chemo treatments will knock the cancer for a loop and give Mom a fighting chance to beat this."

Diane's voice shook with sobs. "It hasn't spread to any distant point, but it has extended locally, beyond the bladder."

"Oh, my God, Mom," Becka, Neil's wife, said. "That's … that's unbelievable. You're fine. You cooked dinner. How did this happen? When did you find out?"

"I had a physical a month ago, and there was blood in my urine," said Diane. "I didn't see it—the lab found it. And it just went from there. A biopsy. A CT scan. A chest X-ray. Lots of tests, and lots of worry and waiting."

"I wish you had told us, Mom. We could have worried with you," said Donna, the oldest. Her voice was chilly.

"Well, Dad and I didn't want to sound the alarm unnecessarily. We wanted some answers before we talked to you girls. Now we have some answers. It's cancer. I'm going to start chemo the day after tomorrow, and then I'll go in for surgery in a few months. I know I'm going to need you girls to help out. I don't know how bad I'll feel, but at least after the surgery, I'm going to need a hand cooking for your father and cleaning this house."

There was a chorus of "We'll help, of course we will." Carl reached for the box of tissues he'd put on the end table right before dinner. "Here. I figured you girls would need these. You always have been criers, the whole bunch of you."

Gail, the youngest, laughed shakily. "Yeah, that's us, the sob sisters." She blew her nose. "What's the surgery all about? To remove the tumor?"

Diane shook her head. "No, it's to remove my bladder. Which is not an appealing idea, but the surgeon said that chances are good they can make an artificial bladder out of my intestine and connect it so I can go to the bathroom normally. If that doesn't work, then it might have to be a little more complicated, with a drain or something. But girls, that's the least of it if I'm healthy afterward, right?"

Gail couldn't imagine her mother, who cared so much about how she looked and what she wore and who always looked fashionably chic, having to deal with emptying a urine bag, internal or external. The whole thing felt sad and . . . wrong.

"Mom, I'm really scared for you. Are you scared?" Gail asked.

Diane nodded and then said, "No, that's not true. I'm not really scared. I'm sad that I might have fewer years to be on this earth than I expected. I'm sad that Dad might be alone, and I'm sad that I might not see the grandkids grow up and that I'll miss good things in your lives. But I'm not scared."

Donna was getting increasingly angry as the conversation continued. Why did they try to do it all alone? Dad driving all the way downtown by himself to take Mom to tests. They're so stubborn sometimes—and who has to pick up the pieces? Us. Me and Becka and Gail, just like when

Dad insisted on taking down the screens himself and fell off the ladder. Who mowed the lawn and took the trash out for weeks?

Finally Donna's feelings erupted. "I can't believe you couldn't trust us enough to tell us before, Mom. I mean, it's kind of a lot to dump on us all at once, you know. Cancer. Surgery. Chemotherapy. At least you could have let us know that you were having tests. How did you think we'd react?"

Diane was shocked by her daughter's anger. But then she remembered what their social worker had told them about people reacting differently to deeply emotional news. Some cry, some withdraw, some experience anger or paralyzing fear. Even so, she hadn't expected any of the girls to lash out. In a small way, she resented Donna's outburst. I'm the one with cancer, she thought. I'm the one who's facing the possibility of wearing a urinary pouch and feeling miserable from chemo. I'm the one who might die. Why should I have to worry about soothing Donna's feelings? She should be worrying about *me*, not turning everything around to make this be about her.

As if she'd read her mother's mind, Donna came over and knelt by Diane's chair. "I'm sorry, Mom. I'm just … freaked. I love you, and I can't stand the thought of you hurting or …"

"Dying." Diane said it for her. Donna nodded. "Hey, don't give up on me so easily. I have every reason to believe that the treatments will cure me. My doctor said I have a 50-50 chance of a cure, and even if the cancer can't be cured, she's confident that treatment will buy me a remission with a good amount of time. I'm going to try not to think the worst, but if it comes to that, we'll deal with it, honey. And I promise that I won't hold back information again."

Carl cleared his throat. "Let's keep in mind that Mom's really going to need us for a while, okay? And," he said in a dramatic voice, "we have something else to talk about."

Gail groaned. "I can't take much more tonight, Dad."

"It's about Thanksgiving," said Diane. "Someone else is going to have to cook the turkey this year."

Chapter 4

Early Stage Bladder Cancer

When applied to urothelial cancer (UC), the word *superficial* can be misleading, and some doctors would like to see use of the term discontinued. Many people equate the word *superficial* with a definition of "not very risky," which isn't always the case.

In general, superficial UC at the low or intermediate risk levels is a highly treatable form of bladder cancer with a good chance for an excellent outcome despite a moderate to high rate of recurrence (depending on the extent and nature of the tumor). But, as we discussed in chapter 3, some superficial urothelial cancers are considered high-risk and carry an elevated chance that the cancer will not only recur, but may have progressed to a more dangerous stage when it does recur.

About 20 percent of people who experience a recurrence are diagnosed with a more advanced type of bladder cancer.

What this means is that superficial bladder cancer, if and when it recurs, will usually come back as a second bout of superficial cancer that can be managed locally. Understanding your prognosis and being informed about the cancer's possibility of recurrence are important parts of your overall treatment process.

Your multidisciplinary team—which may include a urologist, an oncologist, a pathologist, and a radiation oncologist—should welcome your active involvement in your treatment plan and thoroughly explain each step of the process to you. It is worth mentioning that noninvasive bladder cancer is usually managed by a urologist, with support from a pathologist, and typically does not require a full multidisciplinary team unless it recurs repeatedly.

Your treatment plan for superficial UC will include some or all of the following: resection, intravesical chemotherapy, and immunotherapy, which this chapter will discuss in detail, and less frequently cystectomy and perhaps even prostatectomy, which are discussed in chapter 5.

The following descriptions are of a general nature; your experience during your actual medical procedure may differ.

Biopsy and Resection

Most likely at this point you have undergone some of the diagnostic tests discussed in chapter 2. You have had tissue biopsied and classified as superficial UC, and you probably underwent a flexible cystoscopy, during which your doctor thoroughly examined your bladder wall and made a map of the location of abnormal tissue or tumors that other diagnostic tests have confirmed. Sometimes more than one tumor will be present in the bladder, so your urologist will be very careful to look at the whole organ from the inside.

The next step for you is likely to be *resection* (removal of the tumor), unless you've already had a surgical biopsy or rigid cystoscopy. In that case, your doctor may have done a resection to avoid your having to undergo a second surgical procedure under anesthesia.

Undergoing a resection sounds more intimidating than it actually is. Think of it as the removal of the piece of the bladder where the tumor or abnormal cells are growing. This may effectively clear the bladder of tumor, bringing it to a state where only healthy tissue remains.

When you have a bladder resection by means of a cystoscopy, as opposed to invasive surgery, you won't have an incision or stitches, as no external cutting or incision is required.

Resecting (sometimes called *endoscopic resection*) is performed under general anesthesia in a hospital setting. Your doctor will use a *resectoscope*, which resembles a somewhat larger cystoscope. Like a cystoscope, a resectoscope has a lighted lens and is introduced into your bladder through your urethra. (Don't worry; you will be asleep under anesthesia and receiving pain medication while this is happening.)

Your doctor will fill your bladder with water or a non-irritating clear liquid such as glycine, which expands the bladder walls and makes it easier to see tumors and abnormalities. Guided by the map made during the initial cystoscopy, your doctor will use a small wire loop (through which a high-energy electrical current runs) to remove the cancer, a margin of healthy tissue, and a small amount of muscle. Any remaining cells are removed with an electric current or sometimes a high-powered laser. Sometimes your doctor will also take a few random tissue samples from other areas of your bladder to make sure abnormal cells are not developing elsewhere. The tumor, healthy tissue, and muscle are then sent to your pathologist for examination.

A small amount of muscle tissue is included in the tissue sample so the pathologist can verify that the tumor has not spread into the muscle wall. A margin of healthy tissue is removed to decrease the chances that abnormal cells remain in the bladder.

Resection is usually carried out as outpatient surgery. This means that you probably will be able to go home the same day. (You will need a driver to accompany you because you will still be recovering from anesthesia when you are released from the hospital, so you won't be sufficiently alert to drive a car.) You may see some blood in your urine for a few days after a resection, and you may experience pain or stinging when you urinate. The stinging can be eased by drinking lots of fluids and by taking simple pain medications prescribed by your urologist. If either condition lingers longer than two or three days, if other painful conditions occur, or if the bleeding becomes extensive, call your doctor right away.

In some circumstances, your doctor may choose to insert a catheter into your bladder for a short time (usually only one to two days) after the surgery, to prevent blood clots from obstructing the flow of urine and causing discomfort. The catheter allows blood and urine to gently drain out of the bladder and also allows your doctor to irrigate your bladder to promote complete healing of the resected area.

On rare occasions, doctors will recommend another resection procedure. Sometimes the pathologist wants to biopsy muscle tissue from deeper in the bladder wall. And sometimes the tumor is too large to be safely removed all at once.

Sometimes, in an alternative procedure, lasers (high-energy light beams) are used to remove superficial tumors. While patients find this procedure slightly more comfortable than resection, the laser often destroys the tumor tissue, leaving nothing for pathologists to examine. The lack of pathology may limit your medical team's ability to predict recurrence and target your follow-up plan.

If you have been diagnosed with a low-risk tumor, resection may be the only treatment recommended by your medical team. Your team may also recommend a course of intravesical therapy.

Intravesical Therapy

Intravesical means "within the bladder." Intravesical therapy, therefore, is a treatment—in this case a solution containing anticancer drugs—that is administered directly in the bladder instead of being given to you as a pill to swallow or as an injection.

The treatment is given as a liquid poured through an ordinary urinary catheter, the same device that is usually used to drain urine from the bladder. In this case, the flow of fluid is reversed, with the medication being injected gently up through the catheter into the inside of the bladder. Think of it this way: remember when you were a kid and filled balloons with water? If you imagine the bladder as a balloon, filled not with water but with liquid medication sloshing around inside, you'll have a good idea of how intravesical therapy works.

Intravesical therapy has been used for about 30 years as a preventive treatment to reduce the recurrence rate for superficial bladder cancer. It is believed that intravesical therapy works because it destroys cancer cells that may remain in the bladder after resection, thereby reducing the possibility of a recurrence. It also may be absorbed directly into any remaining tumor tissue, thereby destroying the tumor.

There are two types of intravesical therapy, *chemotherapy* and *immunotherapy*, with numerous treatment options within each therapy group.

Your medical team will take a number of things into consideration when deciding which intravesical treatment option is best for you. Their goal is to balance the effectiveness of the treatment with possible side effects and long-term risks based on the type and seriousness of your cancer.

Aggressive treatment options with possibly serious side effects may well be the right choice if you have a type of cancer that has a high recurrence rate and often comes back in a more life-threatening form. On the other hand, if your cancer is low-risk and has a lesser chance of recurring, a more conservative approach might be taken.

Regardless of whether you're advised to undergo a course of chemotherapy or immunotherapy, both are administered

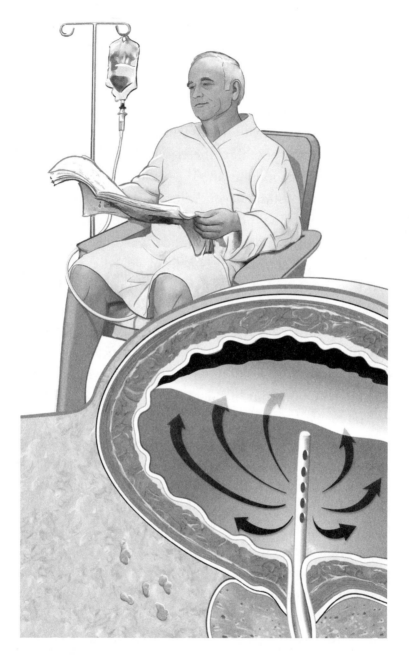

Figure 7—*During intravesical therapy, a solution of anticancer drugs is inserted into the bladder through a catheter.*

the same way. The procedure can be performed either at the hospital about one to seven days after your resection or in your doctor's office if a series of weekly treatments is recommended. The timing depends somewhat on how extensive the resection has been.

First your doctor will numb your urethra with a topical gel and insert a disposable catheter, which will be used to fill the bladder with the solution. The catheter is removed after your bladder is full, and you will be asked to concentrate on not passing urine for a time, holding the solution inside while you get up and move around. Walking, sitting, and standing while the solution is held in your bladder causes it to slosh around and completely coat inside the bladder walls. After an hour or so, you will void the solution just as you would pass urine. In most cases, you will be asked to minimize your fluid intake before the procedure so your bladder won't also be filling with urine that will put additional pressure on your bladder.

The *chemotherapy* drugs that are used in this way include doxorubicin (brand name Adriamycin), epirubicin (Pharmorubicin or Ellence), mitomycin C (Mutamycin), and occasionally thiotepa (Thioplex). Chemotherapy solutions reduce recurrence rates by about 30 percent. However, chemotherapy has little or no effect in preventing superficial cancer from progressing to a more serious stage. What this means is that chemotherapy will often stop the superficial cancer from coming back; however, studies have shown that if the cancer should come back, chemotherapy will not prevent it from coming back in a deeper or more aggressive form. For this reason, the urologist will follow you carefully to ensure that you are not caught unawares by a worsening tumor.

Side effects are fewer from intravesical chemotherapy than from chemotherapy by injection, since a smaller proportion of the chemotherapy drugs gets into the bloodstream during intravesical therapy. Therefore side effects are more likely to be limited to the bladder itself, such as the feeling of having a very nasty bladder infection, rather than affecting the whole body. Side effects after intravesical chemotherapy may also include skin irritation or rash, cystitis (inflammation or irritation of the bladder), leaking of fluid, allergic reaction, and in some infrequent cases a narrowing of the ureters or urethra, making it difficult to urinate. Less commonly there are some "whole body" side effects, such as interference with bone-marrow production (myelosuppression), if the chemotherapy agent is absorbed through the bladder. This usually happens only if intravesical chemotherapy is used soon after resection of an extensive primary bladder cancer, leaving behind a temporarily damaged surface that has blood vessels that can take up the drugs.

Intravesical *immunotherapy* has been used since 1976. *Immunotherapy* means using medicines that stimulate the immunity of your own body (i.e., your immune system) to attack your cancer through the immune response. It is effective in reducing recurrences and in preventing recurrent cancer from progressing to a more serious stage in both superficial urothelial cancer and carcinoma in situ.

A bacterium (a germ or microbe) called Bacillus Calmette-Guérin (BCG) is commonly used for intravesical immunotherapy. This is actually the germ that causes a type of tuberculosis, but it is used in a very weakened or modified form that usually doesn't present any danger at all. BCG works by attracting immune-system cells to the bladder and activating them (turning them "on") to affect the cancer cells present.

BCG Treatments

Bacillus Calmette-Guérin (BCG) is a live bacterial strain in the tuberculosis family. The bacteria are modified so there is little chance of your contracting tuberculosis from the bacteria, but care needs to be taken while you are receiving BCG treatments. Men should sit down to urinate during the six hours after they receive a treatment to avoid splashing urine outside the toilet. About six hours after a treatment both men and women should pour a cup of full-strength bleach into the toilet before flushing. Make sure to wash your hands thoroughly. If urine splashes outside the toilet, wipe it up with a cloth dipped in bleach water and thoroughly wash the cloth (and any clothing that may have been splashed) in hot water.

Although Bacillus Calmette-Guérin is highly effective as an intravesical immunotherapy agent, it has some toxic side effects, and as such is used primarily as a treatment for patients with high-risk types of superficial bladder cancer and those who have had repeated recurrences or CIS.

Side effects may include a burning sensation in the bladder as well as fatigue, chills, and fever. A prolonged high fever and general feeling of being ill may be signs that the bacteria have spread through the body. Because BCG is the bacterium that causes a type of tuberculosis, antibiotics used to treat tuberculosis are usually prescribed when an infection occurs shortly after BCG immunotherapy.

Another type of immunotherapy relies on interferon. Interferon is a protein produced in your body's cells that works much as BCG does to stimulate your body to attack cancer cells in the bladder. Temporary side effects, which usually disappear once interferon therapy is stopped, include muscle and bone aches, fatigue, vomiting, and headaches.

How Much? How Often?

In almost all cases, intravesical therapy (chemotherapy or immunotherapy) is most effective when the first dose is given 6 to 24 hours after resection. Sometimes a single dose is given as a prophylactic (preventative) measure and is not repeated. More commonly, you will receive one dose immediately after resection and then five more treatments on a weekly basis in your doctor's office. In some cases, if a large tumor has been resected, leaving a larger area of ulcerated bladder surface, intravesical chemotherapy will be delayed for a few days to prevent the drug's being absorbed through the damaged surface lining of the bladder. Your doctor may recommend a follow-up cystoscopy after the intravesical treatments are completed.

Keep in mind that there are several types of superficial bladder cancer, some of which have a high risk of recurrence, or progression to a more serious stage. Treatment options, including resection and intravesical therapy, are different for each person and depend upon each person's circumstances.

You may strike up a conversation with another patient in your urologist's waiting room and discover that that patient has had great results and few side effects from a single dose of mitomycin C (MCC) chemotherapy. Even more impressive, he hasn't had a recurrence since his diagnosis three years ago.

You, on the other hand, might be about to undergo your fourth BCG treatment, and each one leaves you feeling as if you have severe bladder irritation for several days afterward. "No side effects and no recurrences" sounds like a better deal than what you are experiencing. So why wasn't MCC prescribed for you?

There could be many reasons. Maybe you have a type of cancer that is high-risk or that responds well to BCG. What you don't want to do is become overwhelmed with worry about whether you're getting the right therapy or whether your doctor is treating your disease properly. Talk to your urologist. Understand your treatment and why it was recommended for you. Having confidence in your treatment plan is very important. Don't wonder about these things. Ask questions!

Other Treatments

On rare occasions, even with a diagnosis of superficial urothelial cancer, part or all of the bladder needs to be removed. If your doctor feels that cystectomy or partial cystectomy (removal of part of the bladder) is called for, he or she will discuss the reasons with you and explain why this approach is preferable to any alternative, less radical treatments that may exist. (See chapter 5 for a discussion of cystectomy.)

What Happens Next?

Apart from giving up smoking, follow-up is the best preventive measure there is for bladder cancer.

For the first two years after treatment, you will undergo cystoscopies, usually every three to four months. If no further tumors are found during that time, follow-up every six months for an additional two years is usually adequate, with annual cystoscopies after that. Because bladder cancer can recur in later years, most doctors in the United States prefer to do annual follow-up cystoscopies for the rest of the patient's life. Some physicians will reduce the number of cystoscopies by alternating them with the urine cytology test (discussed in chapter 2), whereby urine is collected and examined for the presence of cancer cells under a microscope.

Prevention

First and foremost, don't smoke. Don't ride in a car with a smoker. If possible, don't live in a house with a smoker—or at least try to make sure that all smoking occurs outdoors. Become an advocate for living in a smoke-free environment.

Apart from avoiding known carcinogens (cancer-causing substances) and advocating for a general reduction in the use of products known to cause cancer, there is little a patient can do to prevent a recurrence of bladder cancer.

There is some discussion in the medical community about whether routine screening for blood in the urine might lead to earlier diagnosis for people who are at high risk of recurrence. At present, these screening tests are not accurate enough to be completely reliable, but as technology advances, so will the sophistication of such tests, enabling patients to monitor their disease more frequently and with far more comfort.

Many people claim that diet, antioxidants, and various other healthful lifestyle approaches are helpful in the battle against cancer or in retarding the progress of cancer. Frankly, the data are pretty thin, but we believe that it is a good idea to exercise regularly and consume a heart-healthy diet that is low in cholesterol and fats and high in whole grains, legumes, fruits, and vegetables. This doesn't apply only to the battle against cancer; it just makes good sense when you are trying to live a long and healthy life. In light of some of the published medical data, it is probably also a good idea to keep your fluid consumption up, as there is some evidence that bladder cancers occur less frequently in people who have high fluid intake.

What if the Cancer Comes Back?

What happens if your cancer comes back? Most likely, your medical team has prepared you for the possibility.

The signature of bladder cancer is that it can and often does come back, most often during the first two years.

If the cancer does come back, most of the time it is treated just as it was when the tumor was originally diagnosed. You will undergo the same battery of tests or something similar, and the same grading and staging process. And you will probably have the same treatment options, although hopefully, as medicine advances, you will have more and better treatment options available. Of course, if the cancer is more advanced than it was the first time, some differences in treatment will be required. (See chapter 5 for details.)

The key to managing bladder cancer is to tell your doctor promptly if you notice blood in your urine or any of the other symptoms discussed in chapter 1. (Remember, blood in the urine doesn't always signal cancer. It might be there only because of infection.) The earlier a recurrence is detected, the better your chances for a good outcome. Don't wait until your next appointment or decide that you will mention it in six weeks when you're due for your annual cystoscopy. Call your doctor now.

What to Ask Your Doctor about Treatments

The following questions will help you get a clear sense of what will happen during your course of treatment. The questions are only a starting point. Anything else that occurs to you is a worthy question and should be addressed.

What can I expect after surgery? What are the risks of resection?

You may have a catheter in your urethra to help prevent bleeding or blockages. In that case, you may have to stay in the hospital for a day or two following surgery. (When possible, resection is performed on an outpatient basis.) If you are released the same day, your doctor should review possible after-effects such as frequent urination, urine blockage, bladder infection, or blood in the urine and let you know what you should do if you experience any of them. Make sure you ask if there are any restrictions on activity or exercise. Your doctor also should explain any risks, such as blood clots or perforation of the bladder.

What if I have to have intravesical chemotherapy?

Your urologist will administer intravesical chemotherapy, although occasionally patients are referred to a medical oncologist for this procedure. The physician who gives this treatment can give you details about when you will receive the chemotherapy (before or after surgery), how long the course of treatment will be, what side effects you might have (such as bladder irritation or discomfort), and what risks are involved. Make sure you know which members of your team you should speak with if you have questions or concerns about your chemotherapy or about symptoms and side effects of treatment. Your doctor should tell you when to be concerned about side effects and what to do about them (e.g., make an office appointment or go to the emergency room).

What if immunotherapy is prescribed?

There are numerous commercial brands of preparations used for immunotherapy and numerous treatment plans for administering them. You should understand the details of your immunotherapy plan as well as what specific side effects (such as burning or chills and fatigue) are associated with the immunotherapy preparation you will be receiving. Your doctor should tell you which members of your medical team to speak with if you experience problems or have concerns. Your doctor should also tell you when to be concerned about side effects and what to do if a side effect appears (e.g., make an office appointment or go to the emergency room).

When should I come back for a checkup and what can I do to prevent a recurrence? What about screening tests for a recurrence?

Your doctor should schedule a follow-up cystoscopy about three months after your procedure, and he or she should discuss with you if any of the newer screening tests for bladder-cancer markers might be appropriate for you. If you are still smoking, your doctor should encourage you to enroll in a program to help you quit. Your doctor should review the symptoms that might signal a recurrence and discuss what you should do if you experience any of them.

What about having sex? Drinking alcohol? Can I continue to take vitamins or should I stop? How long will I have to be off work? Can I drive?

Ask lifestyle questions as well as any others that concern your personal hobbies or activities. For example, if you love to golf, ask when you can tee off again. If you babysit your grandchildren twice a week, ask when you're likely to feel up to doing so. Do you have a vacation to Maui planned for next month? Make sure you ask if there's any reason you won't be able to go.

Max

Max told everyone that his resection surgery was "a piece of cake." Jean rolled her eyes when she heard him say that and added, "A piece of cake for him, maybe, but he drove the nurses crazy with his jokes."

Humor was Max's way of dealing with the worry and stress. It kept him from thinking about the word cancer.

Max couldn't slough off the worry, though, particularly after his son-in-law started bringing over stacks of information he'd copied from the Internet about treatment for bladder cancer.

"Dad, I know you have a lot of faith in this doctor, but the treatment he's giving you, this BCG, is powerful stuff. I mean, if you splash urine with live BCG on the toilet seat, Mom could pick up the bacteria. She could get TB. So could you. Did this doctor even suggest anything else? Like mitomycin C, for example?"

Max shook his head. "No, he said this BCG was the best for the kind of cancer I have. That's good enough for me, Don."

Max knew that his son-in-law meant well, but all the talk about other treatments was starting to upset Jean.

On the way to Max's next appointment with Dr. P, Jean pulled out a wad of the printouts from her purse and said, "Just ask him about some of this information, okay? Please? I just want to make sure you're getting the right care."

"Fine." Max muttered all the way into the office and was still mumbling about the "stupid Internet" when the doctor came in.

"How are things? Ready to get started next week?" Dr. P glanced at the papers in Jean's hand and knew what was coming. Plenty of his patients had researched their conditions on the Internet and, in fact, Dr. P encouraged them to do so, as long as they were using reputable websites.

"You've been researching," said Dr. P. "Do you have any questions?"

Jean spoke up and explained their son-in-law's concern about BCG. She handed Dr. P the sheaf of articles. He flipped through them and pulled out a couple.

"First of all, let's talk about website information. Some of what you've brought with you comes from good sites that have solid medical information, such as the Cancer.net and the chemocare.com websites. But these," he waved the articles he'd pulled from the pile, "these are from websites that don't update their information and don't have it reviewed by medical experts."

He gave them a checklist and told them how to determine if a website was reputable.

"What about getting TB? That really worries me and seems to be what upsets my son-in-law, too," said Jean.

Dr. P explained that Bacillus Calmette-Guérin is a live strain of the bacterium that causes tuberculosis, but that it's a form that's modified and weakened.

"It's like most treatments, Jean, in that the benefits outweigh—but don't diminish—the risks. But BCG has an excellent track record when it comes to preventing certain kinds of bladder cancer from coming back. Max is at high risk for a recurrence."

They talked some more, even weighing the idea of getting a second opinion, but in the end, Max and Jean decided to go ahead with the BCG treatments.

The doctor gave the stack of papers back to Jean. "You'll have to tell your son-in-law about Quackwatch. He'll like that site."

"What is it? A list of phony doctors?" Max joked.

"Sort of. It's a website, www.quackwatch.org, that exposes health-related fraud, whether it's the sale of untested medicines or websites that don't have good information."

"I love it. For once, I'll have something to tell that son-in-law of mine about the Internet instead of him telling me," said Max.

Max's BCG treatments went well. He experienced some flulike symptoms after each treatment and felt a burning sensation in his bladder that became quite uncomfortable at times, but as Max said, "It was no sweat."

A Few Months Later

Max's first checkup indicated he was clear of cancer. But a few months later, he saw blood in his urine again. He stared for a moment. Then he went out to the porch and gazed out at the lilac bush that had just bloomed.

"I might not see that bush bloom again," Max thought. He knew that the blood might represent bad news. It could mean that his cancer had come back, and this time it might not have such a good outcome. On the other hand, he hoped, it might be just a urinary infection or some sort of late side effect of the immunotherapy.

Max waited until after Jean's birthday the next day to tell her that he'd had a problem. The doctor wanted to do a urinalysis and to see him right away. She, too, knew it might be serious.

When the urinalysis showed microscopic traces of blood in Max's urine, Dr. P scheduled him for an IVP, a bone scan, and an MRI.

"You were right, Max," the doctor said when all the test results were in. "Your cancer has come back, but the good news is that it has not spread outside the bladder."

"What does that mean? Is it curable? Or should I take Jean on a cruise to Tahiti and spend all our retirement money?"

The doctor laughed and said, "No, Max. Better hang onto the retirement fund." A cure was still very possible in Max's case.

"Okay, Doc. What's next? Let's get going and see if we can kill this damn cancer once and for all."

Round Two

First came chemotherapy. This time the drugs were given by injection rather than by catheter. Max went through three months of treatments that left him tired and ten pounds lighter. On one occasion he even had a mouthful of sores that kept him from eating much solid food for a week after the treatments ended.

"Whoever thought I'd hate milkshakes?" Max reluctantly sipped a protein shake through a straw. "If I don't see another milkshake before I die, I won't be unhappy."

Then came the cystectomy, which Max dreaded. The doctor explained that the prostate, bladder, and lymph nodes would be removed. As a result of the surgery, Max would not be able to ejaculate or have an erection. Just as upsetting to Max as not being able to have intercourse was the prospect of having to empty urine from an internal bladder or from an external bag. The mere idea sent him into a blue funk. The doctor's assurances that there were things that could be done about erectile dysfunction and bladder-collection systems didn't help. Max spent a lot of time staring at the lilac bush over the summer, feeling as if everything that made his life worthwhile was slipping away. These days, even his jokes fell flat.

"Well, Jean, you won't be needing those slinky night-gowns anymore, so I was thinking that maybe I'd start buying you power tools for your birthdays instead."

Jean didn't laugh. She said, "Max, I'll just be glad to have you here for my birthdays. I couldn't care less about the sex stuff. Your hugs are all I need."

That was another thing that upset Max. Since the cancer had come back, everyone treated him like a fragile vase that had a crack in it. They talked to him in voices filled with gentle sadness.

One day shortly before he went in for his cystectomy, he blew up at his daughter Nancy and said, "Hey! I'm not dead yet, and I have no intention of dying at all, so quit tiptoeing around and acting as if I'm laid out in my casket in the living room."

Max's outburst cleared the air and the tiptoeing eased up. The cloud of worry and fear lifted a little in Max's heart, too, and he realized that Jean was right: being alive and able to embrace each other was what counted. He was wasting good time by moping around and staring at a lilac bush.

Reconstruction

Dr. P told Max that he was a good candidate for a neobladder, which meant that Dr. P's team would create an internal bladder that connected with Max's "internal plumbing," enabling him to void urine in a normal fashion.

"We may find during surgery that the neobladder isn't going to work for you, Max, in which case we'll do an internal pouch that you manually empty of urine."

The surgery took about four hours, and when Jean saw him in the recovery room, she told him he looked like a plate of spaghetti.

"You've got tubes everywhere! Down your nose, in your side, in your neck ... a urine collection tube ... and heaven knows what else."

Max groaned and drifted back to sleep. For the next four days, he was fed through the nasal tube while he healed. He didn't mind the tube, but he sure got hungry! To his surprise, he was up and walking ... not far, but a few steps ... the day after his surgery, tubes, bags, and all.

Each day Max got stronger and after a few days, the nurses told him to let them know the instant he felt the urge to urinate. Finally it came. He was taking his morning stroll down the hall and had to hurry back to his room, but he didn't mind. He knew it meant that he was healing and the neobladder was working.

One by one the tubes came out and the nurses taught Max how to catheterize himself so he could flush out the bladder on a regular basis.

After 11 days in the hospital, all the tubes were out and Dr. P told Max that he could go home. He took a supply of protective underwear home with him as well as a waterproof mattress pad in case the new bladder leaked.

"Sometimes you'll experience some leakage, Max—especially at night—until you learn to control the process," explained Dr. P. "It's a little different from what you're used to. You have to train yourself to feel things differently and use your muscles differently. Just keep doing your exercises!"

The exercises were nothing more than a series of squeezes in the pelvic area, designed to make the muscles that controlled urination stronger. For some reason Max didn't like doing them.

It took Max a month or so before he felt "back to normal." His appetite was good, he didn't have to take an antibiotic anymore, and his bowels were functioning again. He still needed the protective underwear at night, but he found that he didn't mind it because he was wearing his regular boxers during the day.

Max's first-year checkup was clean. The CT scan showed no cancer. No metastasis. And Max hadn't had any symptoms.

After his second-year checkup, Max stood on the porch, looked at the lilac bush, and smiled. The branches were loaded with blooms ready to burst into flower. Max knew the worry that his cancer might come back probably wouldn't ever leave him. But he finally felt that he could say with some confidence, "I am bladder-cancer survivor."

Living with Cancer

Cancer transforms everyone it touches; many cancer survivors describe their experience as a deep and motivating change. They find that what was normal during their precancer lives no longer applies. Some say that life seems sweeter, that they are embracing life with a gusto and appreciation they didn't have before. Others live with a persistent shadow of worry that their cancer might return, and some are gripped by guilt that they survived cancer while others were not so lucky.

Sometimes cancer survivors are quick to view their personal triumph over their disease as a benchmark for handling anything that might come their way in life, including a recurrence. Others who neither surge with confidence nor shake their fists at fate gradually return to a happier outlook, their faith in their health increasing along with hopes for the future.

Being diagnosed with cancer often gives people the feeling that they have no control. Survivorship is all about learning to take control over how you live the rest of your life.

What can you do to keep yourself buoyed in your evolving role as a cancer survivor? Here are some tips from cancer survivors.

Start or return to an exercise routine. Research has shown that besides the physical benefits of exercise, the chemicals (endorphins) produced by your body during exercise promote a positive outlook.

Eat healthfully. Learning about food and nutrition is easy these days. From websites to magazines and cookbooks to television programs, a wealth of information and countless recipes are readily available. Ask your doctor for recommendations.

Stay connected to life. Survivors say that hobbies, friends, cherished pets, group activities, travel, and social activities get you involved in life.

Stay connected to your spirit. Whether you are religious or not, surviving cancer seems to awaken in many people an increased appreciation for the spiritual. Walking in the woods, listening to the ocean's waves, working in the garden, spending time with your grandchildren, or attending services at your church all nurture your spirit.

Keep in touch with your medical team. While it's not healthy to worry about every ache or pain you experience, knowing when your body feels different is a clue that you need to talk to your doctor. In addition, it's important to follow a regular schedule of checkups—with your oncologist, primary care doctor, and even your dentist and eye doctor.

Take small steps. Sometimes the journey from cancer back to wholeness and health can be slow. Your body, your relationships, even your finances may change during the process. Be patient with yourself and those around you. Let yourself gradually come to the belief that, like Max, you are indeed a survivor.

Walking the Labyrinth

Labyrinth walking is increasingly popular among people who seek a spiritual connection. It's offered in many senior centers, churches, hospitals, and centers such as The Gathering Place in Cleveland, a nonprofit community center for people touched by cancer (www. touchedbycancer.org).

Labyrinth walking can be as simple as following a route chalked on the floor of a community room or as elaborate as a maze constructed of shrubs or stones or room dividers. Regardless of the layout of the

(continued)

labyrinth, your focus is on having a meaningful experience. Many people refer to the labyrinth as a *walking meditation.*

Check with the resource center at your hospital, or ask your social worker or doctor for information on where to find opportunities in your area for labyrinth walking. While this is not a technique of proven benefit, it just might be helpful as an aid to calming you.

Chapter 5

Invasive Bladder Cancer

In the context of bladder cancer, the word *invasive* describes whether cells from your bladder cancer have invaded the muscle wall of the bladder, and if so, how far into the layers of muscle tissue the cancer has penetrated. This can usually be determined from biopsy results, or occasionally when an operation has been performed to remove the bladder and some of the surrounding tissues. In some cases, organs near the bladder (such as the vagina in women, or the prostate in men) may have been invaded as well.

Invasive cancer extends farther into the body than superficial urothelial cancer and is, therefore, a more serious stage of the disease. It requires more complicated treatment, such as surgical removal of the bladder. This may, in turn, change how you manage basic physical functions in your everyday life, such as your bathroom habits and even your sex life. Also of importance is the significant rate of recurrence connected with invasive cancer. Often other organs, such as the lymph nodes, lung, or liver, are involved.

Despite such a gloomy introduction to this chapter, there is every reason for you to be hopeful if you have been diagnosed with invasive cancer. Current treatment, which includes surgery (cystectomy), chemotherapy, radiation therapy, or a combination of these approaches, offers you an excellent chance for long-term survival and, in many cases, for a cure. This applies particularly to those invasive tumors that have not penetrated outside the bladder, the so-called *organ-confined tumors.*

There is no question that the after-effects of surgical removal of the bladder (cystectomy) can be unsettling to think about. You won't have a bladder or maybe even a ure-thra any longer. How will you be able to pass urine? Will you have to have some type of urine-collecting bag? Will there be an odor? Will it show when you wear certain clothing?

We will talk about all those issues in more detail, but in brief, your team will need to surgically create an artificial urine-collection system for you. This is known as a urinary diversion system. In years past, the only option was a urine-collection bag worn outside the body, which many people found to be unpleasant or even embarrassing.

The good news is that now, in many cases, an artificial bladder (sometimes called a *neobladder*) can be fashioned from a piece taken from the intestine (bowel), enabling you to void urine in a normal or near-normal fashion. You will have to learn to use a different set of muscles when uri-nating, and there may be some leakage now and then, par-ticularly at night. Leakage can be controlled by wearing underwear designed with a disposable pad or, for men, a sort of condom. Overall, it's a more attractive option that makes it easier to face a complicated and often scary surgery such as cystectomy. With modern techniques, most patients no longer have to contend with urinary leakage, except on rare occasions.

Even if the creation of an internal urinary diversion system is not possible in your situation, keep in mind that there is also no question that cystectomy is a powerful weapon against invasive bladder cancer that can increase your odds of living a long, cancer-free life.

What Is a Cystectomy?

Cystectomy is the most common treatment option for invasive bladder cancer. In most cases, your medical team will recommend a complete (or radical) cystectomy. This means that your bladder, the lymph nodes tucked around your bladder in the abdomen, the prostate in men, and the uterus, ovaries, and part of the vaginal wall in women will be surgically removed. Depending on where the cancer is located, the urethra may also be removed.

It is easy to confuse some of the terms your doctors use, such as *"cystoscopy* (a diagnostic procedure that introduces a tube into the bladder so the doctor can look at the inner surface and take a biopsy) and *cystectomy* (the surgical removal of the bladder). If you are unsure, don't hesitate to ask your doctors for clarification.

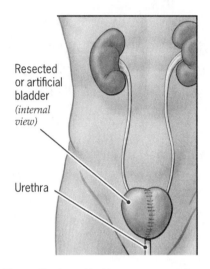

Resected
or artificial
bladder
(internal
view)

Urethra

Figure 8—*A neobladder constructed from the intestine allows normal collection and voiding of urine without manual emptying of a pouch or reservoir.*

Cystectomy sounds like a drastic surgery, doesn't it? Why is it necessary to remove so many body parts? Why not just take the tumor and some surrounding tissue?

Depending on where your tumor is located, the cancer-causing substances responsible for the tumors in your bladder were also filtered through the kidney, ureters, and urethra, and there is a possibility that tumors may be forming in those organs, too. In particular, the tissues lining the bladder, ureters, and urethra (known as the *urothelial tissues*) may be at risk from the after-effects of cancer-causing substances, such as agents in cigarette smoke or industrial dyes. Also, because your cancer may have penetrated the muscle wall, it is possible that organs surrounding the bladder, such as the prostate, uterus, or vagina, may also be at risk of further growth of the cancer cells.

In the case of bladder cancer, which often recurs or spreads to other organs, you will have a much better chance of a cure once organs and tissue have been removed in areas where the disease is likely to spread or where it may already have infiltrated. And a cure, after all, is what you and your doctors are striving to attain.

Sometimes if the cancer is very localized and surrounded by plenty of healthy, noncancerous tissue, a partial cystectomy might be recommended. During this procedure, only a portion of the bladder is removed and some or all of the surrounding organs may be saved.

You probably have already figured out that cystectomy is a surgical procedure performed under general anesthesia in a hospital setting. Depending on what kind of bladder reconstruction you have, you may stay in the hospital anywhere from 5 to 14 days.

The descriptions included here of medical procedures and treatments are of a general nature; your own experience may differ somewhat because there are many different ways of carrying out these procedures.

During a cystectomy, an incision is made through the abdominal wall, so you can expect some mild discomfort at the incision site. The incision will be covered after the surgery is finished, and you probably won't be able to shower or get the incision wet for about a week to 10 days. Your surgeon may have inserted a drain from the incision site, a flexible tube with a hollow bulb on the end that you will remove, empty, flush out, and reattach as needed. Your doctor will remove the drain (a painless procedure) and any stitches or staples in a follow-up visit to his or her office 10 days or so after your surgery.

Cystectomy has some possible complications, including infection, bleeding, blood clots, or intestinal obstruction. You may experience some difficulties with your urinary diversion system. (See the section about urinary diversion systems later in this chapter.) It is also likely that you will have a permanent scar in the abdominal wall—you should ask your surgeon how big that scar is likely to be.

You will be instructed to wait for a few weeks after surgery before you resume driving, and your doctors are likely to want you to refrain for several weeks from doing anything that strains your abdomen, such as pushing and pulling a vacuum cleaner or lifting heavy objects or engaging in any other activity that might damage the scar or even pull the scar tissue apart, thereby risking the formation of a hernia. A hernia occurs when your surgical scar pulls apart under the skin and allows a part of the underlying bowel to poke forward, creating a noticeable lump. Hernias can interfere with the functioning of the bowel and must be repaired, either with an external truss or support, or possibly through another surgical operation. It is smarter to avoid the risk in the first place by not stressing the scar soon after surgery. This is the time to take it easy and, when possible, allow friends or family to pamper you by helping with chores and housework. Just don't get too used to having someone bring you the morning newspaper and a cup of coffee! Generally it is a good idea to review your postoperative instructions with your surgeon so you understand what you can and cannot safely do.

Cystectomy has some negative consequences that you should discuss thoroughly with your medical team. As mentioned above, there may be changes in urinary function. What type of change takes place depends largely on the type of surgery and on whether an artificial bladder has been created.

Sometimes while the abdominal tissues are healing after surgery there will be a period of irregular bowel function, during which you will unexpectedly have to deal with diarrhea or constipation.

Occasionally there will be some swelling in one or both legs, due either to fluid retention or the formation of scar tissue around the lymph vessels that drain the legs.

Often there will be the presence of an asymptomatic, low-grade chronic urinary tract infection that will be identified upon routine testing. This occurs because of the changed pattern of emptying the new bladder. Usually it causes no problems and doesn't require active treatment with antibiotics.

Other issues may also arise. Worries about possible changes in sexual function are common, and very normal. Sexual function often does change after cystectomy. That doesn't mean you can't have an active, playful, pleasurable sex life with your partner. It does mean that you'll probably explore innovative strategies as you seek comfortable ways to experience fulfillment.

Men experience more extreme changes in sexual function after surgery than women do. About half the men who undergo cystectomy experience nerve damage that leaves them impotent after the surgery, a serious lifestyle change that is not only physical but emotional, requiring much thoughtful discussion among you, your partner, and your medical team both before surgery and after.

If you are able to have an erection after surgery, you won't be able to ejaculate, because without a prostate, your body is no longer able to produce semen. You will find that the physical sensation of orgasm is different from what you are accustomed to. It's not unpleasant; just different. In general, the younger you are at the time of surgery, the more likely you will be to have erections or to regain over time the capability of having them. There are surgical procedures, such as penile inserts, that can help make sexual activity possible.

For women, a cystectomy includes the removal of the uterus and part of the vaginal wall. What does that mean for you? Well, for one thing, your vagina may be narrower as a result of the surgery. Usually it is possible to continue to have intercourse, although sometimes there can be some pain involved. Be sure to talk to your doctor if you do experience pain, as there are methods of reducing this.

Most women diagnosed with bladder cancer already have experienced menopause. For younger women, that may not be the case. (Typically, women who receive diagnoses of bladder cancer are older.) The removal of the uterus and possibly of other female organs near the bladder brings an abrupt end to the childbearing years. It may also set off typical menopausal symptoms such as hot flashes or mood swings if the ovaries have been removed at surgery (removal of ovaries is unusual). If you find yourself feeling depressed or blue or uncomfortable from hot flashes, talk to your doctor. You don't have to feel that way; there are options available for you to consider.

As is recommended for men, talking with your partner and your medical team about the physical and emotional changes that you may experience after a cystectomy is an important part of the process, one that deserves as much consideration as the more immediate decisions about which treatment options you want to pursue.

Keep in mind that cystectomy is a life-preserving weapon against invasive cancer. That doesn't mean you can't or shouldn't consider the possibility of impotence or altered sexual function with your partner, or the inability to carry a child. It does offer the hope that you can celebrate many more years of healthy, loving life with your friends and family. That's an important thing to remember at a time when life may seem to be serving you big helpings of despair.

Strategies for Daily Life after Cystectomy

- Drink lots of water. If you have a neobladder or reservoir formed from your intestine, mucus will continue to be excreted from the intestinal tissue and must be flushed regularly to prevent infection. Regular consumption of fluids helps flush out the mucus.

- Maintain good personal hygiene in bathroom habits, hand washing, and/or the care and cleaning of your stoma or reservoir.

- If you have an external pouch, change it daily.

- Learn to recognize the signs of infection, including vomiting, nausea, poor appetite, fever, pain in the back, and strong-smelling or stinking urine.

- Exercise. Did you do aerobics before your cystectomy? Play tennis? Run marathons? You still can. And you should.

- If you're feeling blue, talk to someone. Your doctor, nurse, social worker, spouse, a good friend, and your pastor are all good candidates.

- Take some time for yourself. Listen to music, read a book, take a walk, bake cookies, wash the car, get a manicure.... Whatever relaxes you, make time to do it.

- If your sexual function has changed, don't be afraid to explore different patterns of intimacy. There are many ways to satisfy a partner, many ways to achieve a close and loving relationship. If you and your partner are uncomfortable discussing this side of your relationship, perhaps talking to your doctor or nurse or social worker individually is an option. Whatever your age, you're too young to give up a loving relationship.

- Don't strive for perfection. Just for now, until you've regained your physical strength and the emotional roller coaster has slowed, go easy on the expectations you set for yourself. Let others help, or let the chores go for a while.

Continent Urinary Diversion Systems

Sometimes an internal bladder connected to the urethra (the tube that carries urine to the outside of the body) isn't possible and you will instead be fitted with a continent urinary diversion system. This means that you will have a pouch or reservoir, either external or more commonly internal, that collects your urine, and you will have to empty the pouch. This is also known as an *ostomy* or *ileal conduit system.*

The common continent urinary diversion system is an *internal reservoir,* or pouch, made from a piece of intestine. The pouch is inside your body, but you must manually empty and flush the reservoir by inserting a syringe or catheter into a permanent hole or *stoma* in your abdomen. Often the stoma is located unobtrusively in your navel, where it is not likely to be detected by a casual glance.

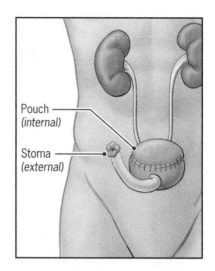

Figure 9—*With a continent urinary diversion system, the urine is collected and stored in a pouch inside the body, and emptied manually through the stoma several times a day.*

Your doctor, may, however, recommend an *external pouch* that is situated outside your body and attaches to your abdomen through a stoma. You must manually empty the external pouch and cleanse the stoma.

Either alternative sounds unpleasant, but having a pouch (particularly an internal reservoir) won't interfere with your life or self-image as much as you might expect, if at all.

You can still snorkel and swim. You can dance in a clingy, swingy dress or bike in Spandex shorts. You can do your job, whether it's manning a drill press or managing a *Fortune* 500 company. And you can still look and feel sexy and enjoy a satisfying intimate relationship with your partner.

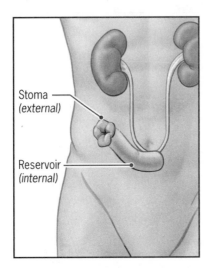

Stoma
(external)

Reservoir
(internal)

Figure 10—*With an ileal conduit system, an external pouch is worn to collect urine and is emptied manually. The pouch connects to the body at the stoma, which empties urine into the pouch as it is collected in the reservoir.*

How is that possible with a pouch of urine attached to your body? Won't it leak or smell?

No, it shouldn't leak, and it won't take you long to adapt to emptying it. Keeping the pouch clean and emptied is the key to feeling—and being—fresh. You'll discover that you can enjoy a glass of wine at a party and excuse yourself a short time later to empty the pouch and freshen up without anyone knowing you have an ostomy system.

External pouches are designed to lie flat against your body and can be discreetly worn under most clothing (even body-shaping underwear for women or athletic supporters for men). Pouches are available in different sizes and with waterproof or protective coverings. Internal reservoirs are even easier to conceal.

You are probably still not convinced that you can look and feel as feminine or masculine as you did without a pouch or reservoir.

For example, what do you do when your partner wants to have sex? What if your pouch leaks or becomes dislodged during an intimate moment? Many patients turn to intimate apparel, some quite sensual, some very practical, that is designed with special protective concealed pockets for your pouch. You can look and feel downright sexy and engage with your partner without worrying. Really.

The Wound Ostomy and Continence Nurses Society maintains a website at www.wocn.org (888-224-9626). The site offers lots of information and a list of apparel companies. One manufacturer is Intimate Moments, on the Web at www.intimatemoments apparel.com (201-825-9931).

Your nurse and doctor can give you tips and instructions. Don't hesitate to talk to them and ask questions. You will want to know what the signs of infection are, whether there are any restrictions on your activities (e.g., some contact sports are restricted), and what diet or exercise constraints you might have.

• • • *Fast Fact* • • •

Certain foods, such as asparagus and some seafood, give your urine a strong odor. You might want to avoid those foods if you're going to be at a party or out in public.
Give yourself time to adjust. Life can be—and usually is—just fine, in spite of having a pouch.

• • •

Treatment Ramifications

Deciding how to treat invasive bladder cancer is a difficult issue for you and your medical team. It is clear that cystectomy can be a life-saving procedure, yet many patients with invasive bladder cancer still eventually die of the disease, especially if the cancer has penetrated the surrounding organs.

Your team will make a recommendation about treatment after carefully evaluating important factors such as the extent of invasion by tumor cells (the stage), the normal or disorganized/abnormal appearance of the cancer cells under the microscope (grade), whether the cancer cells have invaded lymphatic channels or blood vessels, whether cancer cells are growing within the lymph nodes, and whether a specific cell control gene called P53 is normal.

If your cancer is organ-confined (i.e., if the cancer cells have not spread beyond the boundaries of the bladder and its immediate surrounding tissues), if it has not penetrated beyond the first layers of surrounding muscle, if there is no lymphatic or vascular invasion, and if lymph nodes are negative (they contain no cancer cells), the chance of permanent cure by cystectomy alone is about 80 percent.

If, on the other hand, your cancer has penetrated deeply into muscle or has a very poor level of cellular organization (high grade), perhaps if the P53 gene has mutated, or if invasion of lymphatic tissues or blood vessels (*lymphovascular invasion*) is present, the chance of permanent cure may be much lower. If things go badly after cystectomy, the problem is usually that cancer cells show themselves in other parts of the body (*metastases*)—a very dangerous situation.

Over the past half century, doctors have tried many approaches to improve the outcome for patients, including the use of radiotherapy or the combination of radiotherapy and cystectomy. But neither of these approaches appears to have provided the solution. A more proactive approach was devised in the 1970s, when it became clear that cancer-killing drugs (*chemotherapy*) sometimes shrink bladder cancer that has spread through the body, and sometimes can completely eliminate deposits of cancer in different parts of the body. In the past 25 years, studies have looked at the impact of combining chemotherapy with cystectomy or with radiotherapy in an attempt to improve survival figures. Before that discussion, let's talk a bit about chemotherapy.

Chemotherapy

Chemotherapy refers to the use of drugs to kill cancer cells. Chemotherapy is usually given by intravenous injection (injection by needle directly into the vein), but sometimes it can be administered as a tablet or even through a urinary catheter (intravesical) for a patient with superficial bladder cancer (see chapter 4). There are many different types of chemotherapy, and a detailed discussion is beyond the scope of this book. Your medical team will talk with you about what type of chemotherapy is best for you and why.

In brief, chemotherapy drugs mostly act to interfere with the ability of cancer cells to divide and multiply, often by inhibiting the function of enzymes within the cells or by blocking cell division and the formation of RNA and DNA, the substances of life. Because these drugs act on cells that are dividing and multiplying, they can also affect some normal tissues and, therefore, can cause a range of side effects.

Common side effects may include nausea and/or vomiting, hair loss, suppression of the bone marrow (bone marrow forms the blood; its suppression may cause increased risk of fatigue, infection, or bleeding), and occasionally specific reactions to individual drugs (such as allergic reactions and lung inflammation).

Keep your doctor informed if you are experiencing any of the above side effects. Your doctor may recommend additional drugs to minimize these conditions and make your treatment more comfortable. Luckily, side effects tend to disappear once you are no longer receiving chemotherapy, and you will gradually feel stronger and become less vulnerable to bleeding or infections.

For invasive bladder cancer, chemotherapy is sometimes given before a cystectomy. Sometimes it is given afterward. Sometimes it is not given at all. It depends entirely on the type of tumor you have, where it may have spread, and whether you have another medical condition that might make it difficult for you to tolerate chemotherapy. Very advanced age can also be a factor in deciding whether chemotherapy is appropriate.

The choice of drugs used to treat invasive bladder cancer is similar to the choice in advanced or metastatic disease, and we will cover that in chapter 6. If you have invasive urothelial carcinoma, you will probably undergo chemotherapy, because this type of cancer is responsive to either radiotherapy or surgery with chemotherapy, and many studies have examined this type of cancer treatment.

If you have been diagnosed with squamous cell cancer or adenocarcinoma, the outcome for chemotherapy is not so clearly defined. Most physicians don't recommend chemotherapy as *standard* treatment in conjunction with cystectomy for these types of cancer. It is, however, quite reasonable for your team to suggest that you look into a clinical trial (e.g., one that is exploring the use of chemotherapy) if you have been diagnosed with squamous cell or adenocarcinoma. (Clinical trials are not standard care and will be discussed in chapter 6.)

For invasive urothelial carcinoma, most of the information from clinical trials has been obtained from patients who were initially given chemotherapy by intravenous injection and who then went on to cystectomy or to definitive radiotherapy. (More on that later.)

Most of the reported trials indicate that the use of single chemotherapy drugs does not have an extensive beneficial effect, but that the use of combinations of three or four chemotherapy drugs can shrink the bladder cancer in about 70 percent of cases. The drugs can also improve the cure rate and length of survival.

For you as a patient, the information gleaned from these clinical trials means that if you have urothelial cancer, your doctors are likely to recommend treatment that includes a cocktail of several carefully targeted chemotherapy drugs as well as cystectomy or radiotherapy.

With some cancers, such as breast cancer, it is fairly standard practice to give several doses of chemotherapy *after* surgery, especially for tumors with high-risk pathological features, such as lymph-node involvement. We know of six studies that have examined the question of when chemotherapy should be administered for best outcome with bladder cancer, but the results are somewhat inconclusive about whether chemotherapy is most effective if given before or after surgery.

Cares at Cleveland Clinic

Scott Hamilton, an Olympic gold medalist in figure skating, is a survivor of testicular cancer. The experience of being diagnosed and treated successfully for cancer at Cleveland Clinic in 1997 led Scott to dedicate his life to promoting cancer research and awareness.

With Cleveland Clinic Taussig Cancer Institute, he established the Scott Hamilton CARES Initiative (Cancer Alliance for Research, Education and Survivorship) for patients and their families. One of CARES's ongoing projects is the 4th Angel mentoring program, which pairs newly diagnosed cancer patients with people who have been through similar experiences of cancer and cancer treatment.

The CARES program also is the home of www.chemocare.com, Scott's website for people preparing for chemotherapy treatment. The site is jam-packed with tips on how to deal with chemo, how to manage side effects, drug information, and much more.

A large randomized trial is in progress in Europe to study whether intravenous chemotherapy after cystectomy improves the cure rate. Until the results of that study are available, most medical teams recommend consideration of first-line chemotherapy, followed by cystectomy, for deeply invasive bladder cancer. Sometimes a cystectomy reveals a cancer that is deeper or more extensive than had been expected; in that situation, the urologist or oncologist will usually discuss the benefits and drawbacks of using chemotherapy after surgery (called *adjuvant chemotherapy*), typically with the same drugs that would have been given before surgery (see chapter 6).

Some Chemotherapy Combinations and Side Effects

Following are descriptions of some common chemotherapy combinations. This is not an exhaustive list. Talk with your doctor about your treatment plan. Remember that not all people experience all side effects. Your general health, age, other drugs you might be taking, and the dosage of the chemotherapy drugs may affect what side effects you experience. Many side effects are unpleasant, but they are temporary, and the severity of effects is variable. Some side effects are more serious, and you should talk with your medical team about them.

In the bulleted items on pages 122–125 and 127,* represents more serious side effects.

MVAC: Methotrexate, Vinblastine, Doxorubicin (Adriamycin), Cisplatin

This combination of drugs is usually given in four to six cycles of 28 days. The typical treatment is to administer methotrexate on day 1 and vinblastine, doxorubicin, and cisplatin on day 2. Boosters of methotrexate and vinblastine are given on days 15 and 22, and the cycle begins again on day 29. Administration of methotrexate is separated from that of cisplatin by a day, as the two drugs have the potential to interact adversely, causing damage to the kidneys; also, cisplatin sometimes slows excretion of methotrexate through the kidneys. Regular blood tests are made during treatment. If MVAC is used as adjuvant or neo-adjuvant therapy, only three cycles are given in most programs of treatment.

Common side effects, which most people experience, include:

- Fatigue
- Interference with bone-marrow function, which can cause risk of infections, fatigue, shortness of breath, bruising, nosebleeds or bleeding gums, and mouth sores*
- Changes in liver or kidney function (determined by blood tests)*
- Inability to hear high-pitched sounds, ringing in the ears, and/or blurred vision
- Nausea and/or vomiting*
- Possible harm to unborn child and/or infertility, a relatively uncommon problem, as most patients are over the age of 55 years
- Temporary hair loss (usually a complete loss of body hair, which may start about three to six weeks after treatment begins)

- Sensitivity to sunlight
- Pink or red urine for a day or two after treatment

Less common side effects include:
- Temporary irregular heartbeat*
- Redness, stinging, burning, or leakage around the needle/drip site
- Skin rash or itching, dizziness, or headache during treatment (Because these symptoms indicate allergic reaction, you must alert your nurse immediately.)*
- Loss of appetite; metallic taste in mouth
- Diarrhea or constipation (if either continues more than three days, talk with your doctor)
- Tingling or numbness in hands or feet
- Coughing or shortness of breath
- Eyes watery or irritated for a few days after treatment

CMV: Cisplatin, Methotrexate, Vinblastine

This combination is usually given in four cycles of three-week courses. Regular blood tests are made during treatment. On day 1, vinblastine and methotrexate are administered, usually on an outpatient basis. On day 2, cisplatin is administered, sometimes during an overnight stay in the hospital (especially in the case of an older patient or one who is less healthy). The cisplatin dose is higher than for MVAC, and hence doctors tend to use CMV on an inpatient basis more often because of the acute side effects.

Common side effects, which many people experience, include:

- Fatigue
- Interference with bone-marrow function, which can increase risk of infection and cause fatigue, shortness of breath, bruising, nosebleeds, or bleeding gums*
- Temporary hair loss or thinning (this may start about three to four weeks after your treatment begins)
- Kidney damage (determined by blood tests)*
- Inability to hear high-pitched sounds, ringing in the ears, and/or blurred vision
- Nausea and/or vomiting*
- Possible harm to unborn child and/or infertility, a relatively uncommon problem, as most patients are over the age of 55 years

Less common (occasional) side effects include:

- Redness, stinging, burning, or leakage around the needle/drip site
- Skin rash or itching, dizziness, headache during treatment (Because these symptoms indicate allergic reaction, you must alert your nurse immediately.)*
- Loss of appetite; metallic taste in mouth
- Diarrhea or constipation (if either continues more than three days, talk with your doctor)
- Sensitivity to sunlight

- Tingling or numbness in hands and/or feet*
- Coughing or shortness of breath

What is Chemo Fog?

If you are undergoing chemotherapy, you may notice that you have trouble remembering things—even simple things like your telephone number—and you may not be able to concentrate enough to finish your usual morning crossword.

These memory issues, dubbed "chemo fog" or "chemo brain," might be a side effect of the chemotherapy.

Most of the time the brain fuzziness that is a side effect of chemotherapy is short-lived and improves rapidly after treatment ends, usually within six months. But sometimes it doesn't.

Some patients have reported that their cognitive (thought) impairment lasts for months or even years after chemotherapy has ended. And sometimes the fuzziness is more than just forgetting a phone number. It can be an inability to understand basic math or a crippling incapacity to remember how to perform certain tasks, and it can cause great difficulty as you endeavor to carry out duties at work and at home. Fortunately this type of severe problem is uncommon.

Chemo fog seems to be more common in patients who have received large doses of chemotherapy drugs, but researchers aren't sure why some people are affected or how much chemotherapy it takes to cause impairment. Chemo fog is being studied by a number of researchers and is becoming a recognized problem among physicians and patients.

(continued on next page)

Talk to your doctor about any problems you experience with memory or concentration. Your doctor may recommend memory-training exercises and strategies to help your memory or reasoning skills. Some recent research suggests that prescribed stimulants may lessen the effects.

Talk openly with your family, friends, and loved ones about problems you experience with chemo fog. Once they are aware of the problem, you may feel less isolated and inept. As an added benefit, the conversation can open the door for everyone to approach the problem with compassion and a sense of humor.

GEM-CIS: Gemcitabine, Cisplatin

This treatment is usually administered on an outpatient basis. A blood test and saline drip are required before each treatment. The course of treatment usually proceeds in four to six cycles of 21 days (or alternatively on a 28-day cycle), with cisplatin and gemcitabine administered on day 1, gemcitabine only on day 8, with the cycle repeating on day 21. Sometimes an extra dose of gemcitabine is given on day 15, in which case the cycle repeats at day 28.

Common side effects include:

- Risk of infection (contact your physician immediately if you suddenly feel very ill or your temperature goes above 100 degrees)
- Bruising, bleeding, anemia, fatigue

- Nausea*
- Rash, itchiness, swelling in the ankles
- Loss of appetite or food tastes unpleasant; diarrhea
- Tingling or numbness in hands and/or feet*
- Drowsiness*

Less common side effects include:
- Ringing in the ears or other hearing difficulties
- Thinning hair (hair loss is less likely with GEM-CIS)
- Coughing, shortness of breath*
- Possible harm to unborn child and/or infertility, a relatively uncommon problem, as most patients are over the age of 55 years

Radiotherapy (Radiation)

Radiation uses radioactive beams or pellets to kill cancer cells. Your medical team may recommend a course of radiation therapy in addition to chemotherapy and/or surgery.

Radiation therapy for bladder cancer is commonly delivered with a machine that focuses an invisible external beam on the area that requires treatment. The procedure is painless and similar to having an ordinary X-ray done. In the usual approach, your doctors will use your CT scan as a road map of your abdomen and pelvis to pinpoint your tumor and aim the beam at it. In another type of radiotherapy, doctors implant a small pellet or needle of radioactive material directly into your cancer. (This is rarely used for bladder cancer these days.)

When radiation is used alone or with chemotherapy, there is an increased likelihood that your other organs, such as the prostate and uterus, will remain functional, as does your ability to void urine normally and have sex. The intention when chemotherapy *and* radiotherapy are given is usually to improve the chances of curing the cancer while preserving the bladder and avoiding the need to remove it surgically. This area is still somewhat controversial; some physicians believe that this approach is nearly as effective as surgical removal of the bladder, but others feel that cystectomy is the best treatment. The decision of which treatment to pursue depends in part upon the physical fitness of the patient as well as upon the patient's personal preferences.

Radiotherapy is not without side effects. Radiation can scar bladder tissue, and the scarring can reduce the amount of urine your bladder can hold as the bladder wall becomes less distensible. As a result you may experience an increase in the number of times you have to urinate, which can be irritating, especially at night. You also may experience an increase in bouts of cystitis.

There has been much discussion in the medical community about whether the results achieved by radiotherapy are the same as those from cystectomy with respect to achieving cure. We think that when one considers all types of bladder cancer, in the hands of a highly experienced urologist who specializes in this operation, cystectomy gives better results than radiotherapy. However, there are some patients, particularly those with other significant medical conditions, who will benefit from radiotherapy, despite the possibility of a lower chance of permanent cure. In some centers, such as Massachusetts General Hospital, where the techniques of chemoradiotherapy and bladder preservation have been piloted, a urologist will perform a cystoscopy about halfway through the planned course of radiotherapy. If the tumor is shrinking well, radiotherapy will be completed. However, if it appears that the cancer is not responding to radiotherapy, the plan will be abandoned and replaced with a radical cystectomy.

What Happens Next?

There are no absolute guidelines for follow-up after cystectomy. What is right for you will depend on your situation: the type of urinary diversion system you have, whether you received chemotherapy and/or radiotherapy, and what, if any, side effects you are dealing with.

A reasonable guide for follow-up, however, is to expect a physical exam, chest X-ray, urine test, and blood work every three months for the first year, every four months for the next two years, and then twice a year for life. We usually recommend an annual CT or MRI for the first five years at least.

As with superficial cancer, if you have any of the symptoms discussed in chapter 1, check in with your doctor. Call your doctor if you have blood in your urine or an increase in the urge or frequency of urination. It might be an infection, but the best thing to do is to make contact without unnecessary delay.

Because you have an invasive form of cancer, the chance that it may spread to other organs is more likely than with superficial cancer. And the sooner a recurrence or spread (*metastasis*) is discovered, the better the chance of a satisfactory outcome. Therefore, it is important to be aware of any changes in your body and to talk to your doctor about them right away.

Are you more tired than usual—not just today, but on a regular basis? Are you losing weight, even though you are eating more than your share of that chocolate ice cream in the freezer? Do you have any new aches in your muscles or bones, or perhaps a persistent headache?

Even if you have a checkup scheduled within the next few weeks, if you experience any of these signs or symptoms or even just have a vague feeling that something isn't right, don't wait. Call and talk to your doctor.

Prevention

Other than the strategies suggested in chapter 4, there are no specific things you can do to avoid a recurrence or metastasis.

Maintaining a positive outlook—living your life to the fullest without worrying about whether your cancer will come back and whether you will survive if it does recur—is an important approach to dealing with cancer and its after-effects. But sometimes it takes more to achieve this mind-set than just willing yourself not to worry.

To brighten your outlook, activities, interests, and involvements are key. Play with your children, spend time with your spouse and friends, work at a job or hobby you love, nourish yourself through faith or spiritual contemplation, eat well, move and stretch your body as much as you are able, and take time to do at least some of the special things you've always thought about doing, whether it's something as simple as taking a nap on your porch in the sunshine or learning to knit, or as complex as learning to sail. Above all else, *don't smoke!*

Diane

It was Tuesday, day 2 of Diane's MVAC chemotherapy cycle. She dreaded going, not because the process hurt or even because she felt fatigued and a little nauseated for a few days after her treatment, but because it took four or five hours to complete and today was a sunny, midwinter day. It would be so much nicer to be outdoors than cooped up in the clinic, waiting for the intravenous needle to drip.

When she arrived at the clinic, she stopped at the lab for a blood test. Before she could have her chemotherapy treatment, her doctors wanted to make sure that her blood results were within normal ranges. If anything—her kidney-function test, for example—was too abnormal, the treatment might have to be delayed while additional fluids were pushed through to flush her kidneys.

After her blood test, she headed for the chemo lounge to wait while the pharmacist assembled her treatment.

The clinic was crowded and it took about half an hour before Diane's name was called.

"Isn't it depressing to go to chemo?" Carl had asked during their drive that morning to Diane's appointment.

"No. At least not usually. I like to think of it as a place of hope. Without those drugs, I'd have no way to fight this cancer. And I want to fight it."

It was Diane's lucky day. A number of recliner-style chairs were available in the chemo room, and Diane liked the ones upholstered in fabric rather than fake leather. They were softer and not so slippery. Today the blue chair was available—her favorite.

Chemotherapy

Paulette, one of the chemo nurses, threaded a fine tube called a *cannula* into a vein in Diane's forearm. It always hurt a little to have the line put in, sort of like a pinprick, but Paulette started talking about her son, who was trying to decide which college to go to, and before Diane knew it, the line was in.

The doctor had offered Diane the option of a *central line*, a permanent gadget also sometimes called a *port*, inserted under local anesthesia, that would sit just below the collarbone throughout the entire period of chemotherapy treatment. It would spare her the weekly intravenous sticks but it would make showering a bit more complicated. Diane decided to avoid a central line in order to keep things as simple as possible. "I have pretty good veins," she thought, "and hopefully they will be okay for the duration of chemotherapy."

Paulette gave Diane a dose of antinausea drugs through the cannula and then started an infusion (also known as a *drip*) of sterile salt water.

"I wish this part would go faster," said Diane.

"Thirty minutes isn't that long, and it's worth it," said Paulette. "Your kidneys need to soak up a good drink of salt water to keep the cisplatin from doing any damage. Cisplatin is dangerous for the kidneys, so we always flush it through them as quickly as is safe." Paulette patted Diane's hand. "Besides, I taped three episodes of *Monk* for you to watch today. How's that?"

Diane loved Adrian Monk, the obsessive-compulsive detective, and didn't get the program on any of her cable channels at home. Paulette did.

By the time one episode of *Monk* was over, Paulette had finished giving Diane the premedications (antinausea drugs and a type of cortisone to help Diane better tolerate the chemotherapy) and had started administering the vinblastine and doxorubicin. They were colorless, and like the sterile salt water, took a little over half an hour to drip into Diane's system. Paulette was particularly careful when administering the doxorubicin; she had explained that the drug can damage the skin and local tissues if it leaks out of the cannula or if the cannula is not placed properly in the vein.

Then came the cisplatin, also colorless. This drug was administered at a slower rate and took almost two hours to slowly make its way into Diane's body. Diane had taken to kidding that she'd develop bedsores before the cisplatin was done dripping. When the *Monk* episodes were over, Diane tried to read, but as usual, she couldn't, so she closed her eyes and put on her headphones to listen to music.

Finally, after another hour of sterile saltwater (saline) drip, Diane's treatment was over. Paulette slid the cannula out and gave Diane a supply of antinausea drugs.

"You take these—every one, Diane—whether you think you need them or not. You hear me?" Paulette shook her finger. "It's easier to prevent feeling sick than it is to stop it once it gets hold of you." Diane regretted telling Paulette that after the previous treatment she had decided to forgo the antinausea drugs because she felt fine.

Carl was waiting for her in the lounge. "Another one down, baby," she said as she kissed him. "I can feel that wicked cisplatin chewing up those nasty little cancer cells."

Diane knew that she would probably crash once she got home. She hadn't been sleeping well since she started chemotherapy because her feet tingled a lot, especially at night. It felt as if her feet had been asleep and were waking up.

Paulette told Diane that after the treatment ended the tingling would go away gradually over a period of weeks, along with the funny, almost metallic, taste in her mouth. The mouth rinse that the doctor had prescribed helped with the sores in her mouth, but not the funny taste.

When Diane asked whether she was having more or fewer side effects than other patients experienced, Paulette said, "You're about average. Maybe fewer—at least so far. Your hair's getting brittle. That's normal. Some things may get a little worse as we go along."

Diane didn't care what side effects she had or how tough it got. The feeling that the drugs were beating back the cancer gave her the strength to keep going.

She'd be back again, on days 15 and 22 of her treatment cycle, for a boost of methotrexate and vinblastine. Then there'd be a rest before the whole process started over again on day 29.

"Two and a half cycles down, a half to go," Diane said to Carl. "I'll be glad when it's over."

Surgery

Four weeks after her chemotherapy treatments finished, Diane underwent cystectomy surgery.

Diane was grateful that her doctor had spent so much time preparing Diane for what to expect after the surgery. Otherwise, Diane thought, she would have been frightened about the number of tubes and drains and catheters coming out of her body when she woke up. And upset that she was not permitted to drink for a day or two or eat solid food for several days, until her bowel and urinary tract system were back to normal.

Some of the tubes and drains and catheters were connected to the site of the operation and to the internal urine pouch Dr. S had made from Diane's small intestine. The pouch was connected internally to the ureters, which drained urine from the kidneys into the pouch, just as they would into a normal bladder. The difference was that once the pouch healed, it would have to be emptied manually.

For the first few weeks, however, the pouch drained into a temporary external collecting bag through a catheter.

Diane couldn't wait to get rid of the external pouch, but she was looking forward to going home even more. She begged the doctors to send her home a day earlier than planned.

"I just want all these tubes and drains out of my body. My hair is growing back and I want to go home and take a shower, and wear my own clothes, and feel neat and clean and . . . normal."

Deep down, Diane knew that "normal" wouldn't be the same as before she was diagnosed with cancer, but she was determined that no one, not even Carl, would notice anything different about how her body functioned. Emptying and flushing the pouch struck Diane as a messy and distasteful prospect and she didn't want to think about it, much less talk about it.

To her surprise, Diane found that once she got the hang of how things worked, taking care of the pouch wasn't as unpleasant as she expected.

She drained the pouch five or six times a day and once or twice during the night by inserting a catheter into the stoma, or opening, in her navel and letting the urine drain from the internal pouch into the toilet. It took her a month or two to be able to recognize the feeling of the pouch being full of urine and needing to be emptied. It took even longer to learn to thread the catheter into the pouch smoothly and to feel when it was positioned properly in the pouch. The nurse who showed Diane how to use the catheter told her that rolling the tube between her fingers might make it easier to insert, a trick that worked well for Diane. The nurse's advice to relax during the process wasn't quite as easy to follow.

After a few weeks of practice, Diane was able to manage the process well. She knew not to use Vaseline to lubricate the catheter. (But K-Y Jelly was on the approved list and worked very well.) She could tell when she had drained all the urine from the pouch, and she knew how to flush the pouch with saline water once or twice a day. She drank lots of water during the day but reduced her intake in the evening before bedtime. The regular flow of liquid helped control the stoma's mucus production, a natural function since the pouch and stoma were made from intestinal tissue.

Diane even learned a few tricks from talking to other patients in the doctor's waiting room. One woman told her how to protect her clothes from mucus by cutting ultra-thin sanitary napkins in half and taping them over the stoma. The same woman also suggested folding the catheter over on itself and pinching it shut before removing it from the pouch. That way urine wouldn't drain out onto her clothing.

"All in all, I'm managing," Diane told Carl two months after the surgery when he asked her how she was doing. "Better than I expected. I still feel uneasy sometimes, but I guess that goes with the territory. I'm not sure I'll ever feel completely comfortable, but at least I'm over being worried that people might somehow be able to tell that my body works a little differently."

Diane did struggle with anxiety that her cancer would recur, but after her first checkup went well, the worry eased a bit. It eased even more when her second, third, and fourth checkups all were clear.

"Life is good, huh?" said Carl. "We got over the problems early on when it hurt you to make love, and now it's been almost two years and you're still cancer-free."

Diane nodded. "You know, Carl, I don't worry about it coming back anymore, except right before I go in for my checkup. Then I get a queasy feeling and I always worry like crazy until my doctor calls and says it's all good news. Then I go back to not thinking about it. Someone called me a survivor the other day, and it surprised me. I don't think of myself as a survivor, exactly. I think of myself as ... lucky. Blessed with good health and determined to do everything I can to keep myself that way."

Chapter 6

Advanced Bladder Cancer

E ven with prompt and appropriate medical treatment, muscle-invasive urothelial cancer has about a 50 percent chance of *metastasizing* (spreading), either to another organ in the body or within the bladder area itself.

The most common sites of *distant metastasis* (not in the immediate area of the bladder) are the para-aortic lymph nodes and the liver, lungs, and bone. Occasionally, bladder cancer can send deposits through the bloodstream to the brain, but usually this happens only after prolonged and repeated treatment with chemotherapy. Most recurrences, both distant and local, occur within the first two years after treatment.

One point worth emphasizing is that cancer cells in a distant metastasis retain the characteristics of the bladder cancer: they behave like bladder-cancer cells and don't really constitute "bone cancer" or "liver cancer" as such. Therefore, the drugs that may work against bladder cancer cells also have a chance of working against these metastases located at other sites in the body.

As you might expect, the metastasis of your cancer is a dangerous situation that reduces your chance of a permanent cure. But metastasis doesn't mean that cure is impossible or that you no longer have options. Some established chemotherapy approaches can sometimes achieve cure if the metastases are not too extensive. In addition, new and promising therapies, including novel chemotherapy drugs, are undergoing clinical trials as this book goes to print, and many of those may be available to you.

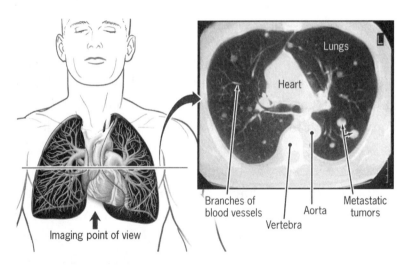

Figure 11—*Imaging can reveal whether the cancer has spread.*

When metastasis occurs, the direction of treatment shifts somewhat away from a complete focus on achieving cure. In this situation, while doctors attempt to cure the metastatic cancer if possible, they also try to *palliate* (reduce) the symptoms, and a greater emphasis is placed on comfort and pain control. This type of treatment is called *palliative care.* At this point, not only you but your family and loved ones should be involved with your medical team, so all of you understand the progression of your disease and are involved in making decisions about your care.

This shift in treatment direction is a very important point and it can be confusing. On the one hand, your medical team is still trying very actively to cure the cancer, if possible, and to prolong your life and improve its quality to the maximum extent. However, because the chance of cure is somewhat smaller, you and your medical team must also give thought to the benefits and drawbacks of treatment, to quality-of-life issues, and to making the decisions that make the most sense. You and your doctors will want to weigh the chance that treatment might be successful against the possible side effects, the time spent in treatment, and the possible limitations on your quality of life.

Your doctor may discover the metastasis during a routine checkup, although sometimes a patient will experience symptoms. It might be bone pain, abdominal discomfort, severe headache, or tingling in the legs. (The latter may occur if a metastasis is pressing on nerves in the spine.) Perhaps you have lost weight without changing exercise or diet habits. A patient might develop a cough or abdominal pain, or experience *hematuria* (blood in the urine) or other symptoms of bladder irritation.

Any of these symptoms should send you to the phone to make an appointment with your doctors. They, in turn, will try to figure out if something sinister is beginning to occur.

As you read this you might be thinking that if the cancer is so advanced—if it has spread to the lungs or bones—what's the point of treating symptoms such as tingling in your legs or vague abdominal pain?

Doctors take these symptoms seriously because even though the cancer has advanced and metastasized, you are likely to live for an extensive period of time—months or years—and it makes good sense to make sure that you are able to live that time as comfortably and as fully as possible. If symptoms go untreated, your ability to participate in everyday life with your family and friends may be greatly diminished, and the time you have left with them may be cut short.

On the other hand, *occasionally* a specialist may decide to watch and wait. A doctor might make this choice, for example, when a change is seen on an X-ray but the patient is not experiencing any other symptoms. Or when a patient is unwell from other medical problems or is just keen to avoid treatment at that time. In such situations, sometimes the decision will be made to observe closely and start treatment when symptoms occur.

What kind of treatment can a patient expect if the cancer metastasizes? Surgery to remove the bladder is occasionally a possibility if the only site of recurrence is the bladder and surrounding tissues. It usually doesn't make sense to operate if the cancer has spread to distant sites.

Sometimes radiotherapy will be used to reduce the symptoms of recurrence in the bladder if the recurrence is too extensive to permit surgery or if distant metastases have also occurred.

Chemotherapy is usually used if the cancer has spread widely or to distant sites, and radiotherapy is sometimes used for an isolated metastasis (for example, to the brain or to a bone). A palliative care specialist may be brought in for consultation on how to reduce your pain or make you more comfortable as your disease progresses. And your doctors may talk with you about participating in a clinical trial. (We will talk about clinical trials later in this chapter.)

For the most part you can expect to remain at home, with any treatment taking place on an outpatient basis. There are exceptions. You might require a short hospital stay to manage a particular symptom, such as resistant pain or a bowel obstruction, but the goal is to keep you at home, with your family, participating in as much of life as possible.

Chemotherapy

As mentioned in the previous chapter, current practice is to blend chemotherapy drugs to get a head start in treating the cancer before it becomes too extensive. The goal is increased effectiveness in fighting advanced bladder cancer. This practice has often resulted in a longer and more comfortable life span for many bladder-cancer patients and has made it possible to offer increased hope.

A quick review: *Chemotherapy* is a term that refers to drugs that fight cancer, usually by causing cancer cells to die or causing the process of their growth to stop. It is often a liquid medicine given by injection into a vein. Sometimes it can be administered as a tablet. Chemotherapy treatment is usually provided on an outpatient basis, although certain drugs, such as cisplatin, may be given during a short inpatient stay.

Chemotherapy treatments—which drugs are given and how often—vary from person to person, depending on the stage of disease, the patient's age and overall health, and many other factors. Usually you will receive the drugs intravenously (by needle into a vein), and each treatment will take from one to several hours. You may receive several treatments over the course of a month, and treatments may be given for up to six months or occasionally a bit longer. (More information about chemotherapy is available in chapter 5, including a detailed discussion of side effects and potential benefits.)

Chemotherapy has many uses. It is given to reduce or eliminate cancer cells present in your body, as well as to prevent existing cancer cells from growing and flourishing. Chemotherapy can inhibit and sometimes prevent the formation of new cancer cells. It can shrink tumors so that they are safely operable. When chemotherapy is used to stop bladder cancer from coming back after treatment by cystectomy or radiotherapy, it is called *adjuvant therapy*. Chemotherapy is not yet able to cure all cancer, but it has certainly opened the door for many people to enjoy many months of extended life.

Chemotherapy is powerful medicine. In addition to damaging cancerous cells, it can damage cells in the bone marrow that produce blood cells. This means that your blood count may be lower than usual. A shortage of white blood

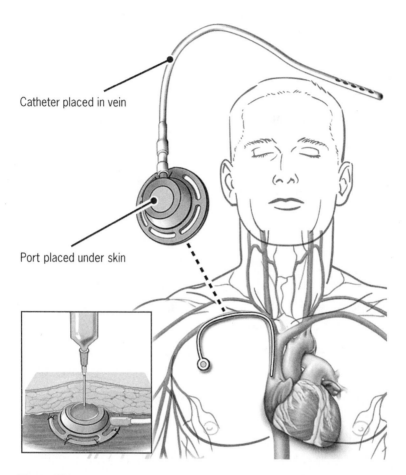

Catheter placed in vein

Port placed under skin

Figure 12—*Chemotherapy can be given through a surgically implanted port. The tail of the port is positioned in a vein so the chemotherapy drugs can be delivered directly into the bloodstream. Only a portion of the head of the port (where the chemotherapy is injected) is accessible outside the body. The port remains in the body until treatment comes to an end.*

cells can leave you vulnerable to infections. A low platelet count may lead to bruising or even extensive bleeding from minor cuts and scrapes. Low red blood cell counts leave you feeling fatigued or exhausted (a condition called *anemia*).

These side effects usually go away after the treatment concludes. Temporary symptoms such as nausea and vomiting can be controlled to some extent by drugs, while other, more permanent side effects can occur, such as infertility or premature menopause.

Developments in the Use of Chemotherapy

There are many chemotherapy drugs or agents, and it has been known for 50 years that some of these can cause advanced or metastatic bladder cancer to shrink or even disappear. The problem is that sometimes the cancer will recover and start to grow again.

Although many anticancer or chemotherapy drugs have been shown to work against advanced or metastatic bladder cancer, the list in routine use today is somewhat smaller. Before describing the different drugs, it is worth mentioning that a series of clinical trials (see pages 150–162 for a discussion of clinical trials) has shown that combinations of chemotherapy drugs administered together are *usually* more effective than the use of single drugs. For many years, a combination of four chemotherapy agents (methotrexate, vinblastine, doxorubicin (brand name Adriamycin), and cisplatin), the so-called MVAC regimen or treatment, has been used as a standard chemotherapy for advanced bladder cancer. Some years ago, a trial demonstrated that MVAC gave higher shrinkage rates and longer survival than cisplatin alone and that it was also superior to a regimen that combined three drugs (cyclophosphamide, Adriamycin, and cisplatin).

The problem was that the drug combination was quite toxic, with side effects that included nausea, vomiting, a sore mouth, risk of infection, and occasionally problems with cardiac (heart) function. Despite the problems, about 60 to 70 percent of patients experienced shrinkage of their

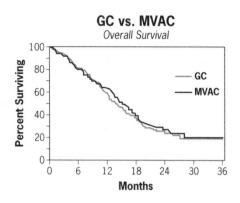

Figure 13—*A comparison of two chemotherapy regimens routinely used for bladder cancer shows that the survival rates are similar.*

metastatic bladder cancers in response to this treatment, and there were patients who survived in good health for several years after such treatment (without recurrence).

Investigators with an interest in bladder cancer have collaborated with scientists to try to find less toxic and more effective drugs than the three-drug regimen. Between 1985 and the present time, several new drugs have been identified, including ifosfamide, paclitaxel, docetaxel, and gemcitabine. In a series of clinical trials, each of these drugs showed some activity against advanced bladder cancer. The two that have been most frequently incorporated into modern treatment approaches are paclitaxel and gemcitabine. As single drugs, each has been shown to shrink cancers that have previously received chemotherapy (and have recurred), and they have both been shown to be active against previously untreated cancers.

Today, one of the new standards of chemotherapy for bladder cancer is a combination of gemcitabine and cisplatin. This combination has been shown to cause tumor shrinkage in around 60 to 65 percent of cancers and to sustain survival to an extent similar to that of the MVAC regimen. In fact, a trial conducted by the Eli Lilly Corporation (the company that makes gemcitabine), with participation by cancer specialists around the world, specifically examined the combination of gemcitabine and cisplatin in comparison with the MVAC regimen. The proportion of patients surviving in each treatment group was very similar, but the gemcitabine-cisplatin combination was much less toxic than MVAC. As a result, many cancer specialists now view gemcitabine-cisplatin as a new standard of care for patients with metastatic disease. It should be emphasized that a similar randomized clinical trial has not been completed for patients who need neo-adjuvant or adjuvant chemotherapy, and thus the standard in that case remains the MVAC regimen.

Not resting on their laurels, the clinical research community has moved forward and is now testing a new combination that adds paclitaxel, another active drug mentioned above, to the gemcitabine-cisplatin regimen. A three-drug combination (gemcitabine-cisplatin-paclitaxel) has been compared to the two-drug standard, to see whether this produces better cancer shrinkage and improved survival. In June 2007, the first report of this trial was made public. It indicated that the three-drug combination offered no significant benefit compared to gemcitabine-cisplatin and was associated with more side effects.

Another new agent, pemetrexed, also targets the division and reproduction of cancer cells, and has a relatively gentle profile with regard to side effects. Pemetrexed is being tested in patients who have already been treated with gemcitabine and cisplatin to see if it causes tumor shrinkage. Early reports are promising, but the drug's real usefulness is not yet known with certainty, and it has not yet been assessed by the U.S. Food and Drug Administration, which must give formal approval for its use in the treatment of bladder cancer.

In addition to the use of chemotherapy, another class of anticancer agents, the so-called growth inhibitors or targeted agents, is being tested in patients with advanced bladder cancer. It is known that proteins located on the surface of cancer cells can control the rate of DNA production and division and stimulate cancer-cell growth. An example is the epidermal growth factor receptor (EGFR), which sits on the surface of some bladder-cancer cells and helps to control the rate at which they grow and divide. Inhibitors of the function of EGFR (and of the genes that control its production) have been developed and are known to slow or stop the growth of some cancer cells. The agent Herceptin (generic name: trastuzumab), for example, has shown anticancer activity in breast cancer, another type of malignancy in which EGFR plays an important role. Trials have been completed in which EGFR inhibitors such as Herceptin have been combined with chemotherapy, and preliminary analysis suggests the possibility that the combination of Herceptin and chemotherapy may improve results. This is being tested in further clinical trials, to verify that this is a true advance and also to discover if there are hidden costs (such as unexpected side effects) associated with the drugs.

Most recently, preliminary data suggest that a new class of anticancer agents, the tyrosine kinase inhibitors, may also be effective against bladder cancer. For example, the agent sunitinib (brand name: Sutent) has been shown to shrink bladder cancers. This agent helps to inhibit *angiogenesis* (the formation of tumor-supporting blood vessels) by interacting against a system of enzymes (tyrosine kinases) within the cancer cells that stimulate cancer growth and blood-vessel production. More information will be required before these drugs become a standard of care, and many clinical trials are testing this concept.

Clinical Trials

A clinical trial is a research study designed to test how well a new drug, therapy, device, or treatment works for people. The trial is an experimental research process conducted according to strictly regulated scientific and ethical principles that require people who participate in these trials to receive close medical supervision. A clinical trial can *only* be conducted if the patient has been given detailed information about the trial, both written and verbal, and has been given the opportunity to ask questions about benefits and drawbacks to participation. In addition, all clinical trials are reviewed independently by institutional review boards (IRBs), which consider the ethics of the study, the safety of patients, and whether the research is actually worth doing. The protection of patients' privacy is also an issue that an IRB will oversee, so information about trial participants is not disclosed inappropriately.

A clinical trial may include fewer than 100 people monitored at just one or two locations, or it can involve thousands of people monitored by many doctors, nurses, data collectors, and other researchers at diverse locations such as doctors' offices, hospitals, clinics, or medical centers.

Clinical trials are sponsored by government agencies such as the National Cancer Institute, as well as medical institutions, individual doctors or other medical personnel, medical foundations, and drug companies or companies that manufacture diagnostic testing equipment.

Some Benefits and Risks of Participation in a Clinical Trial

Possible Benefits

- During a trial you will receive thorough medical monitoring and attention from doctors and other health professionals
- If your cancer is resistant to treatment or has recurred, clinical trials offer another treatment option
- You will receive high-quality cancer care, and if you are in a test group for a new protocol, you may be among the first to benefit from a new treatment that has the potential to be highly effective
- You have the opportunity to help other cancer patients by contributing to the improvement of cancer treatment
- Your participation in a trial may enable you to feel positive and proactive about your treatment plan

(continued on next page)

Possible Risks

- Your health insurance may not cover all your costs
- The monitoring requirements of the clinical trial may demand more of your time than a nontrial treatment would
- The new treatment being tested may not prove as effective as standard care
- There may be increased or unexpected side effects
- The treatment you receive, whether it is a standard-of-care treatment or a new treatment being tested, may not work for you

---

You may be alarmed if your doctor suggests the possibility of participating in a clinical trial. Does it mean that you have no hope? What should you do? How should you respond?

It is important not to dismiss the idea out of hand. The words *experimental, research,* and *human volunteer* can be upsetting, particularly at a time when you are dealing with the emotional issues surrounding a diagnosis of advanced cancer. But treatments in clinical trials can often be highly beneficial to the patients who volunteer. You and your loved ones should talk with your medical team members about the clinical trial they are recommending and why it may benefit you. Noteworthy to many patients is that several studies have documented that patients who participate in clinical trials have better outcomes than those found in the community at large. However, this also may also be due to the types of patients who agree to participate in trials.

Does referral to a clinical trial mean that there is no hope of your surviving this illness? Not at all! There is always hope of survival, and any doctor can tell you about people who have responded positively to treatment and not only survived, but thrived. Participating in a clinical trial doesn't mean that you won't continue to receive medical treatment; you will, and since the trial is a voluntary process, you have the right to stop participating in the trial at any time.

As with any aspect of your treatment plan, you make the decision about whether to proceed. Don't feel pressured to participate in a trial if it doesn't feel right for you, but do give it objective thought and consideration.

How do you begin weighing the pros and cons of whether to participate in a trial?

Probably the first question that comes to your mind is whether clinical trials are safe. Scientists and medical investigators work hard to ensure that they are as safe as possible. The medical community and the U.S. Department of Health and Human Services have rules in place to ensure that every clinical trial is highly regulated and reviewed by health-care professionals, who determine that the trial is designed and conducted in compliance with federal regulations governing research on human volunteers. Everything about the trial, from the doctors involved to the people who volunteer and the treatment being tested, is subject to strict review and monitoring. However, it is important to understand that some clinical trials *do* carry increased risks.

As with any treatment, you should ask about possible risks, benefits, and side effects, how the treatment works, and what results doctors expect from the study. You will want to know who is conducting the clinical trial and what kind of oversight is in place. Also ask what is expected of you. Where will you go for the treatments? How often will you go? Are there more tests or office visits than you might have with standard treatment? Who administers the treatments and how are the results measured? Do you have to report regularly to the people who are conducting the trial? Who pays for it all? Will there be extra costs to you as a result of your participation? Will the team conducting the trial (or the doctors involved) stand to benefit personally from the results of the trial or its conduct?

Types of Clinical Trials

There are many kinds of clinical trials. Some test *prevention*, such as whether vitamin C prevents colds. Some test whether particular *screening* tests, such as mammograms for breast cancer, are effective. The clinical trials your team is likely to mention are *treatment* trials, whereby a new drug, a new treatment, or even a new way of applying a standard treatment will be examined and tested.

Each treatment trial will have a very detailed and specific plan called a *protocol*. Think of a protocol as a recipe or instructions that describe what will be done in the trial, why the trial is necessary, who is eligible to participate, and how it will be conducted. Any doctor or researcher who takes part in the trial uses the trial's protocol to ensure consistent results and to make sure that the new drug or treatment is given properly and with maximum safety.

Within treatment trials, there are four categories, or phases. You should ask the members of your medical team which phase of clinical trial they are recommending to you and find out specific details about the trial, such as the number of people involved, where the testing is being done, what benefits or drawbacks are expected for you personally, and how long the trial is expected to last.

Phase I trials study how to administer a new drug or treatment and how much of the drug or treatment can be safely tolerated. The drugs or treatment in a phase I trial have been extensively tested in a lab and in animal studies, but not in humans. If a drug is being tested, researchers may start by giving a very low dose of the drug to those participating in the trial, then increase it gradually to determine when side effects appear and what dosage is tolerable, yet effective. Phase I trials usually enroll a small number of people at a limited number of locations. In general, they are the least likely to be of direct personal benefit to a patient, as the drugs are less well known, but occasionally they can lead to significant tumor shrinkage with side effects well within the tolerable range.

Phase II trials take the studies a step farther. From the phase I results, researchers know what dosage to give with a good margin of safety; in phase II they are ready to test whether the drug really works as well as anticipated. They carefully monitor patients in the study for side effects and observe closely how the drug affects the cancer. A phase II study usually targets a particular disease or type of cancer and includes fewer than 100 people.

Phase III trials involve large groups of people across a broad geographical area. A random process determines which individuals will receive the drug being tested and which ones will receive standard treatment. The idea is to compare accurately whether the new treatment is better than the old treatment and whether there are different patterns of side effects and survival. The results are monitored closely, and if one treatment is observed to be significantly more effective than the other, the trial is stopped. Sometimes a phase III trial will find that the new treatment is not better than the standard, in which case the new treatment is usually dropped from the list. Studies are *randomized*—patients are chosen randomly for the new and standard treatments—to avoid introducing biases into the study. For example, without randomization, there might be an inadvertent tendency to choose younger and stronger patients for the new agent and older patients with other medical problems for the established treatment. This might make the new treatment appear to be better than the established treatment when, in fact, the differences were attributable only to the type of patient receiving each type of treatment. In some cases, where the benefits of a new drug are really uncertain, and it is not clear whether the new drug is better than no treatment at all, a phase III trial will compare the new drug to a placebo (an inactive agent). This is done to exclude the possibility of patients experiencing perceived benefit just because they are receiving treatment itself, rather than because the drug is actually reducing the cancer. As surprising as it seems, this effect (known as the placebo effect) really does occur occasionally. Doctors are required by law to inform patients if they are using a placebo in such a trial.

Phase IV trials typically take place after the drug or treatment has been approved for standard use. The trial may include up to several thousand people whose medical progress is monitored while they are receiving the drug or treatment. Results are logged to determine how well the drug or treatment is performing in the real world (in other words, in a series of doctors' offices and clinics rather than in the setting of a specific clinical comparison trial).

Many trials, particularly phase III trials, bring together an independent committee of medical professionals, patient advocates, and statistical researchers in a body known as a Data and Safety Monitoring Board (DSMB). The DSMB oversees the trial to ensure that there is no unexpected pattern of serious side effects, that tumor responses are occurring with a reasonable frequency, and that patient welfare is protected. Of course, as previously mentioned, clinical trials cannot occur without approval from an independent or institutional review board (IRB), which reviews the nature, risks, and benefits involved.

Before you are enrolled in a clinical trial, you will need to meet the eligibility requirements spelled out in the protocol. Eligibility requirements help researchers make sure that results are consistent and that your participation in the trial won't make your condition worse. What kinds of criteria constitute eligibility requirements? Researchers may want people within a specified age range who are a specific gender and who share particular characteristics pertaining to their medical situation and current health. For example, the

Questions to Ask About Clinical Trials

- What is the purpose of the trial study and who is sponsoring it?

- How long will it last?

- Who is monitoring the study? What results are expected?

- How will my safety as a participant be ensured?

- What do I have to do if I participate?

- What procedures or tests are required?

- What are the risks and benefits to me?

- What side effects might I experience?

- What costs will I have to pay? How much will those expenses be?

- What will my insurance cover?

- What other options do I have regarding my treatment?

- What about new medications? Will I be able to continue to take my regular medications?

- Who will be my doctor? Who is in charge of my care?

- Where will the study take place? Do I have to travel, and if so, who pays?

- Will the study affect my daily life? How?

- Can I drop out at any time?

- Compared to standard care, will there be extra costs or extra risks?

- Do the physicians involved in the trial have any conflict of interest? Do they receive payment for conducting the trial? Are they shareholders in the pharmaceutical company that provides the drug?

clinical trial that your doctor recommends to you may be for men between the ages of 60 and 85 who have bladder cancer of a particular type and stage and who have never previously received chemotherapy.

Institutions Conducting Clinical Trials

Recent clinical trials on bladder-cancer treatments (as of October 2009) have taken place or are in progress at the following locations:

- Cleveland Clinic Taussig Cancer Institute (clevelandclinic. org/cancer)
- Memorial Sloan-Kettering Cancer Center, New York, New York (www.mskcc.org)
- M. D. Anderson Cancer Center, University of Texas, Houston, Texas (http://mdanderson.org)
- University of Michigan Comprehensive Cancer Center, Ann Arbor, Michigan (www.cancer.med.umich.edu)
- University of California, San Francisco, San Francisco, California (http://medschool.ucsf.edu/research)
- Dana-Farber/Harvard Cancer Center, Boston, Massachusetts (www. dfhcc.harvard.edu)

A reputable place to start looking for current information on cancer centers pursuing clinical trials is the National Cancer Institute's comprehensive clinical trial center (http://cancercenters.cancer.gov). You'll find information there about the cancer centers conducting clinical trials along with links to their websites.

A document called an *informed consent* will help you sort through your questions and concerns. The form, which you sign, includes a disclosure statement from the researcher describing the protocol, who is conducting the trial, what tests will be made and how, the possible risks and the possible benefits to you, and what side effects are anticipated. Informed consent gives you information you need to make a decision about participating in a clinical trial. An informed consent states that you agree to participate in the clinical trial and requires your signature.

Signing an informed consent form does not mean that you are legally bound in any way to remain in the clinical trial. You may drop out at any time. Before the trial starts, after it's under way, during the follow-up period—anytime.

Informed consent doesn't end once the clinical trial has begun. Researchers are obligated to tell you if they find new side effects, benefits, or risks to participating in the study.

Who Pays?

You have decided to participate in a phase III clinical trial in which a new drug is being tested by a research team. Who pays for it?

Your usual care costs—those you would incur whether you are enrolled in a trial or not—are usually covered by your insurance plan or Medicare.

But the extra care costs that are incurred by your participation in a clinical trial may not be covered. Often if a drug is being tested, it is provided to trial participants free of charge. But you may have a side effect, such as nausea, and require an antinausea prescription to address the complaint. Your insurance company may view the antinausea medication as an extra care cost. The clinical trial may or may not pay for the antinausea drugs or other office visits or tests specifically required as part of your being in the trial. Sometimes federal funding or grant programs help pay the costs; sometimes they don't.

If neither the trial nor federal programs cover the cost, you or your insurance company will be expected to pay.

Sadly, your insurance company may or may not agree to pay costs for expenses associated with the clinical trials. Some insurance companies consider such treatment experimental and, as such, refuse to pay. Before you agree to participate in a study, contact your insurance company to determine what your plan covers. Some states have passed legislation requiring insurance companies to cover the costs to patients of clinical trials. Federal health insurance, for the most part, covers clinical trials. Medicare does, for example, and so does health insurance through the Department of Veterans Affairs and the Department of Defense. Things change, however, and you should double-check your coverage before going ahead with a clinical trial.

If your insurance company does not cover clinical trial expenses and you want to participate, ask someone from your medical team or the clinical trial team to contact a representative from your insurance company. Sometimes after claims representatives review the clinical trial protocol, they will approve payment. Also, the National Cancer

Institute is working with many health-insurance and managed-care providers to find answers to the question of how to provide coverage for clinical trial participation.

The National Coalition for Cancer Survivorship offers a publication entitled *What Cancer Survivors Need to Know about Health Insurance* that helps patients navigate the financial maze. You may order the publication at the organization's website (www.canceradvocacy.org/resources/publications) or call 877-622-7937 to request a copy. The National Cancer Institute's *Facing Forward: Life after Cancer Treatments* includes a section on insurance issues. It's available at www.cancer.gov or you can order it by calling 800-422-6237 (800-4-CANCER).

An extensive list of resources, websites, and helpful publications that deal with a wide range of subjects, including insurance and financial assistance, is available in appendix B at the back of this book.

After a clinical trial is over, the results are often published in medical magazines or scientific journals. Once a new drug or treatment has been deemed effective and safe, it becomes standard practice; this means that doctors accept and use the drug or treatment while providing everyday medical care.

The National Library of Medicine has links to the results of many clinical trials at www.nlm.nih.gov.

Chapter 7

When Things Don't Work Out

E nd-of-life decisions are difficult, painful, and heart-breaking. They raise issues we don't want to face, either for ourselves or with someone we love.

Yet at times, despite aggressive and thorough care, there are no further drugs or therapies or surgeries or clinical trials with curative possibilities, and the only option a patient's medical team has to recommend is hospice care.

The goal of hospice care is not to cure disease; its goal is to provide palliative care—comfort, pain relief, and support—for those facing end-of-life choices. Hospice care addresses quality of life. It involves a team approach similar to the medical team model. Hospice providers offer palliative care specific to people facing an end-of-life diagnosis and their families.

Hospice care does not mean that a patient won't take any more medications or that there may not be some continuing therapies to help with symptoms and quality of life. In the case of advanced bladder cancer, it means that a patient's medical team has determined that further medical strategies are not likely to cure his or her bladder cancer and are not likely to prolong life. Death is the likely outcome, and the emphasis of treatment will change to focus on control of symptoms.

Death. It's such a hard word. Such a scary concept.

The questions pile up in patients' minds. Will there be a lot of pain or indignity? What about being physically able to enjoy the rest of life? How to take care of the overwhelming, ongoing business of life? What about a funeral? What about family? Whom to tell? How to deal with the outpouring of sympathy and questions from family, friends, church members, coworkers? What about cost?

And the emotions pile up in patients' hearts. There's the reality of missing so much in the rest of life. The anger and grief about Why me, why now? The last time to savor spring's gentle bloom or a grandchild's birthday. Coming to terms with the inevitability of death. The good-byes.

These are the sorts of practical, medical, personal, and emotional issues that a hospice-care team can help with. Let's look at how this process works through a series of questions and answers.

Questions and Answers

What is the difference between palliative care and hospice?

Palliative care is a broad term that describes a supportive approach to treating anyone dealing with a serious or life-threatening illness. Someone who has AIDS, for example, may benefit from palliative care. Palliative care focuses not on curing a patient's medical situation, but on providing comfort and relief from suffering during or after treatment. Most hospitals have a palliative care team that is separate from hospice. The palliative care team helps with symptom control for patients who are receiving treatment and may recover from the cancer.

Hospice is a specific, defined type of compassionate palliative care offered to patients facing an end-of-life diagnosis. There are private hospice organizations, both for-profit and nonprofit; in some cases, hospitals have an in-house hospice team. Hospice care can be administered at a patient's home or in a medical setting such as a hospital or nursing home.

At Cleveland Clinic, Taussig Cancer Institute's Harry R. Horvitz Center for Palliative Medicine and Cleveland Clinic Health Care Ventures, Inc., are among the available options for palliative care or hospice services.

Why all the talk about pain management? Other than my back starting to ache now and then, I'm doing okay.

A new or persistent pain, whether a nagging backache or a shooting pain, can signal that a patient's cancer has changed or grown in some way. Doctors depend on patients to

166 · The Cleveland Clinic Guide to Bladder Cancer

describe any pain, however intermittent or insignificant, so they can better treat not only the disease, but any affiliated pain as well.

For example, a tender, aching pain in the upper back or shoulder *may* indicate that cancer has moved into the chest cavity or bones. A patient might feel a squeezing cramp in the abdomen or a shooting pain that feels like an electrical current. It is important to remember that the presence of a new pain doesn't necessarily mean that cancer is active at that site, as pain can be caused by many other factors, such as infection or inflammation.

Each type of pain tells doctors something different and requires a different combination of drugs and therapies to help minimize discomfort while managing the progression of the disease.

Some people resist telling their doctor about pain because they think that pain management involves using drugs such as morphine that leave patients pain-free but occasionally in a drowsy fog, and they don't want to spend their days "doped up." Some people fear the possibility of addiction, even if they are dying.

Because of the many options available today to control pain, these problems usually don't occur, although the first few days of pain medication (before the optimal dose is found) may be associated with some drowsiness or nausea.

There may be circumstances when narcotic drugs such as morphine are the best option for pain relief. But usually doctors can combine non-narcotic anti-inflammatory or nonsteroidal anti-inflammatory drugs (such as ibuprofen) that will do the trick, leaving patients alert and able to participate in some of the things they love to do, whether sewing or baking apple pie or even golfing. There can be side effects from these drugs, such as nausea, shortness of breath, or itching, athough most are either temporary or can be controlled with other drugs.

That's not to say that a patient's days will be a constant round of taking pills and more pills. Some medications are easily absorbed through the skin from a patch or a suppository. Other medications can be injected at regular intervals or even dispensed through a pump (usually implanted under the skin).

Additionally, not all pain relief relies on drugs. Radiation therapy can relieve some types of bone pain, and doctors can surgically block a nerve's pathway, interrupting the transmission of pain signals to the brain. Acupuncture or electronic nerve stimulation are still other ways of managing pain.

Years ago, doctors held off prescribing drugs for pain until the pain was unrelenting. Those days are long gone, and doctors today subscribe to the theory that no one's life should be interrupted by severe pain of any sort. With all the options available for pain management today, most of them nonintrusive and without significant side effects, there is no reason for anyone to endure even minimal pain.

I'm feeling well and am still active and involved in my life, even though my doctor told me that I probably only have a year or so to live. Why did she recommend hospice care already?

A medical team is likely to suggest hospice care when there are no drugs or therapies left that are likely to cure a patient's disease or significantly prolong his or her life and when emotional or spiritual comfort and care are needed. Most doctors recommend that patients begin thinking about hospice when an end-of-life diagnosis has been made, so that they can begin discussing and making decisions about their care and wishes.

Hospice offers an interdisciplinary approach that extends past medical services to embrace and coordinate professional services from many disciplines. A hospice team typically includes a patient's personal doctor, a hospice physician, nurses, home health aides, social workers, clergy, counselors, other therapists as needed, and a core of trained volunteers.

The hospice team coordinates all aspects of a patient's care: medical needs, medications, pain, help at home, bereavement counseling, help in a hospital or nursing-home setting, and support for emotional, psychosocial, and spiritual aspects of dying. The hospice team also supports a patient's family and loved ones.

How do I get into a hospice program? Where do I find one?

Anyone can call a hospice provider and ask for help, although in most cases, a referral is made by a doctor. In either case, a physician must certify eligibility for hospice services. Eligibility generally means that a patient has been diagnosed with a terminal illness or condition with a life expectancy measured in months rather than years.

A doctor, senior center, or hospital can probably provide a list of local hospice programs. The National Hospice and Palliative Care Organization also provides help through its website at www.nhpco.org and by phone at 800-658-8898. Medline Plus has a state-by-state list of providers at http://medlineplus.gov. In Ohio, referrals are available through www.hospiceohio.org.

Choosing hospice does not mean giving up hope. It does mean choosing a strategy to maximize quality of life while stabilizing a patient's medical condition and getting practical help in planning a comfortable, supported, and pain-free end of life. Sometimes facing the prospect of death overpowers the remaining gifts that life has to offer. Hospice eases some of the burdens—financial, medical, and emotional—and offers opportunities to savor each sunrise, each crisp apple or juicy peach, each hug from a friend or loved one, and the gifts of laughter and love and memories.

Who pays for hospice? My insurance? Me?

Medicare and most private insurance companies pay for hospice expenses. Most hospices are certified by Medicare, and most people who use hospice are over 65, the age of general eligibility for Medicare. The Medicare Hospice Benefit, available to people with Part A Medicare, pays for virtually every cost associated with hospice care, from medications to counseling services.

Most insurance companies have provisions for paying for hospice benefits for those under the age of 65. However, hospice programs certified by Medicare are required to provide a specific set of core services to anyone needing hospice care regardless of insurance.

Hospice benefits do not cover any ongoing medications or therapies prescribed for cure rather than comfort.

What is hospice? A place?

It can be. Some hospice providers have private care facilities, but in most cases, hospice is provided in a patient's home, in the hospital, or in a nursing home. Hospice is a type of service, not a place.

What if I don't like hospice? Am I stuck?

No. A patient can leave hospice at any time and reinstate regular health-care benefits and care. Conversely, a patient can go back to hospice at any time, provided that he or she remains eligible. Hospice benefits can remain in place indefinitely, although a patient must periodically be recertified as eligible.

There are lots of hospice programs around. How do I know which one is best?

Asking for recommendations from health-care professionals, nursing homes, clergy, senior centers, or trustworthy people who have used hospice services in the past is a good way to start. The National Hospice and Palliative Care Organization (NHPCO) maintains a helpline at 800-658-8898 (and a website at www.nhpco.org) that can provide assistance as well. The organization has a comprehensive tool called "Standards and Practices for Hospice Programs" that is complex but offers detailed information on how hospice programs should be structured and should handle specific concerns.

What should I ask a hospice agency?

Before making a choice, interview the hospice agency. Below are some questions to get you started:

- What services are provided?
- How involved will my doctor be in my care?
- What support services are available to me and my family, and how do we take advantage of them?
- How many volunteers do you have? What kind of training do they get? What sort of services are your volunteers involved in?
- What happens if something is needed outside normal business hours?
- Is your program certified by Medicare?
- What if in-patient care is needed? How is it handled?
- What about pain? What do you do for comfort?
- Who will be on my interdisciplinary team? How many families does the team care for at once? How often will the nurse visit?
- Do you ask families to complete a satisfaction survey, and if so, may I see the results?
- Are you accredited by any professional organizations? Do they perform periodic inspections, and if so, may I see the results?
- What happens if I can't stay in my home because of increasing care needs?
- Who pays for this, and is it mostly covered by insurance?

Do I have to sign anything such as a living will?

Hospice providers believe in death with dignity, and they affirm death as a natural, normal process. As such, hospice respects patients' goals, preferences, and choices as long as those choices neither prolong life through active anticancer therapy nor hasten death. In most cases, patients receiving hospice care choose to sign *advance directives,* documents designed to tell family members and medical professionals what kind of care should be provided if and when the patient is no longer able to make such decisions.

One type of advance directive is a *living will,* a legal document that describes what kind of life-sustaining medical treatments you want, if any. A second document, a *durable power of health care (*sometimes called a *health care proxy* or a *medical power of attorney),* lets you identify the person you want to make health-care decisions for you, if necessary. A *Do Not Resuscitate (DNR)* document instructs medical professionals not to perform cardiopulmonary resuscitation (CPR) or other life-saving efforts if you stop breathing or your heart stops. These documents are legal in most states, and your doctor's office or hospice team can tell you where to get forms. Online forms and a description of advance directives are available through the National Hospice and Palliative Care Organization site (www.nhpco.org), which links to www.caringinfo. org/AdvanceDirectives. Information can also be found at the AARP site (www.aarp.org/research/legal/advancedirect).

In keeping with the hospice philosophy "neither hasten nor postpone death," many hospice organizations ask for a signed DNR; they may or may not require other advance directives.

What You Need to Know about Living Wills

- A living will lets you determine in advance and *while you are able* what kind of medical care you want if you are *unable* to express your wishes because you are terminally ill or permanently unconscious. (If you are able to tell your doctor what care you want, a living will cannot be invoked.)

- Laws governing living wills vary from state to state. Check with your state government or an attorney to determine what is required. Websites with information on state laws include: http://estate.findlaw.com/estate-planning/living-wills.html and www.caringinfo.org. Your living will gives your doctor(s) the authority to allow you to die naturally, without life-sustaining treatment other than that necessary to make you comfortable or to relieve your pain.

- In your living will, you have the choice of *giving* or *not giving* your doctor the authority to withhold food administered through a feeding tube. You decide in advance whether you want your life extended if the time comes when you require such artificial means of life support.

- The law requires your doctor to make every effort to notify your closest relatives if your living will is invoked. Your closest relatives have the right to legally challenge the doctor on whether your medical condition is such that your living will should be invoked, but no one can legally challenge your right to determine for yourself whether you want or do not want your life extended by artificial means.

- A living will cannot be enforced if your family, persons holding powers of attorney, physicians, or caregivers don't know about it. Make sure your loved ones and

(continued on next page)

health-care professionals who provide your care (including hospital officials) have a copy of your living will.

- You may revoke your living will at any time by informing your doctor of your intent. It's a good idea to ask for any copies of your living will to be returned to you, and you should destroy the copies.
- Your living will takes precedence over a health-care power of attorney. A living will takes effect when you are permanently unable to express your wishes; a health-care power of attorney designates someone to make health-care decisions for you if you are temporarily unable to do so yourself.

How long does it take for hospice care to start?

In most cases, hospice care starts almost immediately after a referral is made. Typically, a hospice worker will meet with a patient and his or her doctor within 48 hours and begin working on a plan of care that includes among many other things an evaluation of the services and medications the patient or loved ones might need. Some of the options might include a medication plan or a referral to a grief group or cancer support group.

I don't know whether hospice is right for me. I'm feeling hopeless about what's facing me. Where can I turn for support?

For a careful and candid discussion about your choices and expectations, your doctor is often a good place to start.

Cleveland Clinic's toll-free Patient Resource Cancer Answer Line (866-223-8100) is another good option, especially if your doctor seems reluctant to discuss such matters. Two cancer nurses are available to answer questions and provide resource help on weekdays between 8 A.M. and 4:30 P.M. (You don't have to be a Cleveland Clinic patient to call the Cancer Line.)

Many support groups are available for cancer patients and their families and friends. Cleveland Clinic's social work department (216-444-6552) or the Cancer Answer Line mentioned above can help you find a group that meets your needs, as can social workers at the hospital where you are receiving treatment or the American Cancer Society (800-227-2345 or www.cancer.org). The American Cancer Society website also has public message boards for people who wish to participate.

At the downtown campus at Cleveland Clinic, the Patient Resource Center at Taussig Cancer Institute is open weekdays from 8 A.M. to 4:30 P.M. The Resource Center offers brochures about cancer, listings about support groups and resources, and computer terminals for Internet searches.

The National Cancer Institute's Information Service (800-422-6237 or 800-4-CANCER) can provide help to patients and their families who need to locate programs, services, or resources.

The Visiting Nurse Association of America (www.vnaa. org or 888-866-8773) can provide resources for skilled nursing, mental-health care, hospice care, or home health care.

Caregiver Stress

In families grappling with an end-of-life diagnosis, the patient is not the only one having a rough time. Sometimes the people who are caring for loved ones with cancer don't pay enough attention to taking care of themselves. They are so focused on the daily responsibilities of providing good care to the person who is ill that they overlook their own need for rest and food and exercise.

How do you know when you have crossed the line from good care-giving to caregiver stress?

One hallmark is that you can't go to sleep, or if you do, you are restless. Because you aren't sleeping well, you feel tired and burned out all the time. That fatigue can lead to being irritable and short on patience. You start to feel like a zombie, doing things by rote and without enough attention, or perhaps you resent having to do so much for someone else and feel guilty about feeling resentful. You might eat too much, or not care about eating at all. Maybe you've started to drink a second—or third—glass of wine.

Any or all of the above can be signs that you're not taking enough time to take care of yourself.

You're probably shaking your head and thinking, I know that. But what can I do to change it? Someone has to be there night and day, giving medication and baths and changing the sheets three times a day.

You're right. Someone does have to be there. But perhaps it doesn't always have to be you. Can you afford to have a home care worker come in for a few hours once a week? If not, is a friend, relative, or neighbor able to relieve you? If you can't work something out with a paid home care worker or friend, talk to your doctor or social worker. There are options.

Once you have an hour or two for yourself, how do you spend the time? Don't feel guilty about taking a little time for yourself. Think of it as recharging yourself so you can go back to your caretaking duties refreshed and alert.

Choosing a Home Care Agency

Here are a few questions to have handy when you are looking for home care for yourself or a loved one:

- Is the agency licensed by the state? Certified by Medicare? Accredited by a national organization such as the Joint Commission on Healthcare Accreditation?

- How long has the agency been providing cancer care? Does the agency provide the services you need or expect you will need? Does the agency own or can it arrange for equipment that you (or home care staff) might need?

- How are home care workers hired, trained, supervised, and monitored? Are they licensed?

- Who bills Medicare and insurance, you or the agency? Who follows up on claims?

- What happens if you need emergency care? What happens if a home care worker doesn't show up? Is a 24-hour contact available?

- Does the agency have a patient's rights statement? Is it available for you to review?

- Do you feel comfortable talking with agency personnel? What if you have a complaint?

- Can the agency provide references from current clients?

You probably have a long list of errands to do, and your first thought may be to fill those free hours by going to the dry cleaner, the hardware store, or Target. While it's fine to drop off a pair of shoes for repair while you're out and about, do reserve this time to do something *refreshing*.

Go to the library and sit in a quiet corner to read. Get your nails done or have a massage. Go out to lunch or play nine holes of golf with a friend. Go to the gym or recreation center and have a swim and a sauna. You get the idea—do something for *you*.

Even if you can't get away for a short time every day, there are things you can do to ease the daily stress. Buy a yoga DVD to use at home or indulge yourself by watching a favorite television program. If you like to read, why not read a book aloud to the person you are caring for, or pop some corn and watch a movie together? Finding ways to smile and laugh each day makes a big difference, too.

If you are able, join a caregiver support group. Not only will it help you feel refreshed, but you might learn some great tips about being a caregiver and find some sympathetic shoulders to cry on when the going gets tough. These days, online support groups make it possible to connect with others even when you *can't* get away.

Do be cautious in joining online groups, however. You might want to read the article "How to Find an Online Support Group" at the American Cancer Society's website, www. cancer.org. The ACS has its own online support resources at its Cancer Survivors Network, www.acscsn.org.

Cares for Caregivers

Olympic gold-medalist and cancer survivor Scott Hamilton learned firsthand how scary cancer can be for both patients and the loved ones responsible for their care, and he decided to do something about it. With Cleveland Clinic Taussig Cancer Institute, he established the Scott Hamilton CARES Initiative (Cancer Alliance for Research, Education and Survivorship) for patients and their families. From this, the 4th Angel mentoring program for caregivers was born. This national program pairs mentors who have been caregivers with new caregivers who need firsthand answers to some very hard questions. Mentors and caregivers meet by phone or through e-mail; all you need to do to be paired with a 4th Angel mentor is to call 866-520-3197 or visit www.scottcares.com.

Tim

For four or five months, Tim hadn't been feeling himself. He'd been tired, for one thing. Really tired. He started taking a multivitamin, thinking that he might be low in iron, but it didn't seem to help. He tried fixing himself healthier meals, but half the time he'd scrape most of what he cooked down the disposal. Nothing much tasted good anymore.

Then he started noticing spots of blood in his underwear. He figured he had a kidney problem. Maybe a kidney stone. That would account for the persistent dull ache in his side, too. He bought a jug of cranberry juice but before he could drink it all, the spots of blood became a daily thing and he decided he'd better call his doctor and get things checked out.

"You've lost eleven pounds since the last time you were here," the nurse announced after she weighed Tim. "You'd better stop dieting. You're getting a little too skinny."

"I'm not dieting," Tim said. "I don't have much of an appetite these days, that's all."

After examining Tim, Dr. L asked a lot of questions about when Tim had noticed the spotting and the ache in his side, and whether he felt any pain in his lower back.

"What do you think is wrong?" Tim asked. The serious look on the doctor's face worried him. Tim had been coming to Dr. L for a long time, maybe 15 years, and the doctor usually joked and asked Tim about where he'd been fly-fishing lately. Today Dr. L was all business.

"I think we need to do some tests, Tim. A CT scan, a urinalysis, and a bone scan, for starters."

"A bone scan? That's not good, I know that." Tim buttoned his shirt. "Look, just tell me what you think is going on. I'll only imagine the worst if you don't."

Dr. L explained that while he didn't want to jump to any conclusions before he got the test results, he suspected that Tim was seriously ill.

"The bones in your lower back are tender, your liver is enlarged, you've lost weight, and you've experienced intermittent hematuria, or blood in your urine," said Dr. L. "I suspect either a serious infection or possibly cancer, but we won't know for sure until we get the test results."

As soon as the word was out of Dr. L's mouth, Tim realized that he'd been worrying about cancer ever since the nurse pointed out how much weight he'd lost. Tim knew that a significant unintended weight loss was potentially a sign of cancer.

The Follow-up Appointment

When Tim came in for his follow-up appointment after his tests, Dr. L sat behind his desk, papers arranged neatly in a pile in front of him, hands folded. Not good news, thought Tim. If it were good news, he'd smile.

Instead, Dr. L straightened some papers and started talking in a calm, low voice. Each word he spoke added to Tim's fear and worry. Large deposits in the liver. Blood in his urine. Spots of cancer on his rib bones. Bladder cancer that has spread to other parts of his body.

"So what do we do about all this?" asked Tim. "What kind of treatment? There's so much you can do these days for cancer."

"Well, I'm going to refer you to an oncologist at the Taussig Cancer Institute for the answer to that question, Tim. We'll work as a team, but for advanced cancer treatment, you need a specialist."

"How soon can I get in?" Now that the diagnosis of cancer was certain, Tim felt as if he had to do something. Right then. Get the cancer out or start doing something to kill it. He couldn't just sit still and wait for appointments.

"As long as it takes us to cross the street," said Dr. L. "One of the clinic's oncologists is working out of the Strongsville satellite campus today, and my nurse arranged for her to meet with us this afternoon."

Before the two men left the office, Tim said, "You know, I've been coming here a long time, since before my wife died. You can be straight with me. How bad is it?"

"That's a question we need to ask the oncologist," said Dr. L. "Bladder cancer isn't my specialty, and whatever statistics I give you are likely to be outdated or flat-out wrong. But I can tell you it's serious, Tim."

Tim nodded. "Okay. Fair enough."

Aggressive Treatment

The oncologist was direct with Tim. "We're going to do an aggressive regimen of chemotherapy with gemcitabine and cisplatin, drugs that have a proven track record against bladder cancer. It's a manageable regimen, Tim. You'll probably experience mild nausea and fatigue and perhaps tingling in your feet. And there's risk of infection. I can give you some medications to help with the side effects but they won't be alleviated entirely."

Tim nodded. He appreciated the doctor's frankness in explaining what lay ahead of him.

"With this aggressive regiment of Gem-Cis, we have a 40 to 60 percent chance of shrinking the cancer."

"Wow, that's a better cure rate than I expected," said Tim.

Dr. L and the oncologist exchanged a somber look.

"What was that look about?" Tim asked." Is there something you're not telling me? Look, I can handle this if I know what's going on, what to expect. What I can't handle is uncertainty and worry."

"That's fair, Tim, and I'll try to meet your expectations." The doctor cleared her throat. "There is always hope for a cure, but we cannot be sure. At this stage of advanced cancer, Tim, your chances of a permanent cure are less than 10 percent. What you need to keep in mind is that while the chemotherapy may not cure your disease at this point, it may stop any further spread of the disease and hopefully, result in a remission (or tumor shrinkage) that might last for months or even years. Your chances of a remission are about 40 percent."

Tim sat quietly for a moment. The odds weren't as good as he'd hoped. But someone had to be among the 40 percent who had a remission. Tim would do everything possible to make sure he was one of them.

"I can deal with those odds," he said. "It's almost even-steven. You just tell me what I need to do to help myself be one of the 40 percent, and I'll do it."

Tim had a rough time with the chemotherapy, but he refused to give up or lose hope. And indeed, he turned out to be one of the lucky ones. He went into remission after his Gem-Cis treatment and for 14 months spent every available moment with his son and two grandchildren.

"These babies are better than chemotherapy," he kept saying. "And fewer side effects, too."

Then, just after his 72nd birthday, Tim felt an ache in his gut. He ignored it for a few days, but when it didn't go away, he went back to see his oncologist, who ordered a round of blood tests, a bone scan, and a CT scan.

Tim knew the news wouldn't be good, and it wasn't. His cancer was back. It was in his liver and bones again.

His doctor told him that it was time to consider two things: a clinical trial and hospice care.

"I don't much care for the idea of being a guinea pig," said Tim. "But if I can help find a better treatment or a cure for this disease, then I'll do it."

"I'm going to refer you to a social worker, Tim. She'll help you through the process of deciding about a clinical trial, and she'll get you some information about hospice."

"I'm not ready for hospice," Tim said. "Maybe down the road, when I'm not doing so well . . ."

His doctor said, "I think you should think about it now. I know you're not ready, but it's much easier to get the paperwork done now and get to know the people that you'll be working with in hospice now, before it's a crisis situation. It's hard to let outsiders such as hospice caregivers into your family at a private time like this, Tim, but I don't think you'll be sorry. Hospice can make a big difference."

His doctor gave Tim a brochure about a phase II cancer trial under way at Cleveland Clinic.

"I'll talk to my son. We've already talked about this a little, and he's all for me doing what I can to help the research efforts. He's an optometrist and knows how much research has benefited his field," said Tim.

"I remember you telling me that about your son. I hope you'll take part, Tim, but if you don't, that's okay. Clinical trials aren't for everyone. Some people want the reassurance of being treated by their doctor at their hospital. Others get a lift from helping research efforts."

The Cancer Progresses

Tim's cancer progressed more quickly than anyone expected. Within four weeks, the pain in his back and abdomen had returned. Sometimes it was quite intense. He was glad he'd taken his oncologist's advice and let his social worker set up hospice care for him. He just didn't feel like struggling further, and he changed his mind about the clinical trial.

A nurse and hospice social worker came to his house a few days after his appointment with his oncologist. They explained how hospice works and talked about the hospice philosophy of care.

"Our goal is to help create a place of rest and comfort for you and your family," said Nancy, Tim's hospice nurse. "We provide comfort care and make sure your pain and symptoms are under control so you can live your life with as much gusto as possible and even fulfill some of your life wishes. We offer a team approach to meeting your spiritual, physical, and emotional needs. And we try to help you accept the process of dying while embracing life. It's a complex emotional time, one that can bring fear, hope, worry, grief, sadness, joy, anger, and eventually, peace."

The hospice social worker helped Tim put in place a living will and a durable power of health care. Tim didn't want to prolong his life with any breathing machines or feeding tubes, so he talked to his social worker about signing a Do Not Resuscitate (DNR) order.

Tim showed his son the documents and explained that he wanted to die as peacefully and painlessly as possible. It was a sad afternoon, and the two of them shared not only tears but laughter. They looked at old pictures and videotapes, drank

Tim's favorite root beer, and ate a whole plate of peanut-butter cookies that Tim's neighbor had brought over.

It wasn't too long before Tim started feeling enough pain that his hospice team suggested a regimen of medications and massage therapy for him. They arranged for a hospital bed and for a home care worker to cook and clean for Tim a few times a week.

"It's amazing what these people do for me, how much they care," Tim told his son. "They make this whole thing bearable and manageable, and believe me, sometimes it's just so overpowering that I can't think or function. I wouldn't have known where to turn or what to do without them."

Tim sat quietly for a minute before continuing. "You know, sometimes in the middle of the night hopelessness gets the best of me and I feel so alone in the darkness, so afraid. I mentioned it one time to Nancy when she said the black circles under my eyes looked like bruises. And you know what she did? She gave me a number I can call any-time, day or night, to talk to someone in hospice. I never have called. Maybe because the comfort of knowing I *can* call helps get me through the night."

"Dad, you can always call me, anytime."

"I know, son, but you're dealing with your own emo-tions about all this. I hate to lean on you too much. I like it that our visits are mostly talk about the kids and what they're doing and everyday things. It makes me feel normal, and that's nice."

Once the symptoms were brought under control, Tim decided to consider the clinical trial again. He was adamant about wanting to participate. Nancy, the oncologist, Tim, and his son sat down to talk about it together. They hashed over whether the regimen of medication and follow-up care would be too much for Tim, and talked about whether the possible side effects might impair the quality of his life.

"Will this be a benefit or a burden, Tim?" asked Nancy. "Is it worth it?"

"You bet it's worth it," said Tim. "It's probably too late for me to benefit from this trial, but you know, maybe someday my son or someone else's son will be diagnosed with bladder cancer. And I'd like to think that if that happens, there will be a new and promising treatment available … and that I helped make that possible."

Tim's son hugged him. "Dad, you are an incredible man."

"If I were so incredible, I would have stopped smoking years ago. The day you were born. But the fact is, I wouldn't want to do this if you hadn't inspired me, son." Tim took a pen and signed the consent forms for the clinical trial. "I've come to feel that doing this means that my life will be remembered in some small way. As if I'll participate in creating a legacy for future generations, and there will be a breath of my spirit in those who benefit from the research. That's a bit of peace and comfort I didn't expect from all this. And you know, I might be one of the lucky ones and respond to the treatment, right?"

When Tim stopped speaking, there wasn't a dry eye in the room.

Coping with Grief

Grief is about loss. It may be your grief about losing the rest of your life to cancer. It may be your loved ones' grief about losing you to cancer. Either way, emotions during the grieving process are varied—from shock, sadness, worry, and guilt to emptiness, anger, or fear—and the feelings come and go with amazing speed.

Maybe you can't concentrate on anything, even something as familiar as writing checks to pay bills. Maybe you wake up a lot at night or have bad dreams. You may not care about cooking meals, let alone eating them. You may cry a lot or feel numb, or experience what seems like unending waves of sadness.

It may not seem like it, but all those emotions and feelings are not only part of the grief process, they are part of the healing process as well.

Here are some things you can do to work through the grief process.

Be with people. Friends, family, loved ones. Let them buoy your spirits and ease a bit of your pain.

Do normal things, even though sometimes you might not feel like it. Go out to dinner with friends. Plant your garden. Clean the house. Get a pet. It's okay to do these things; it doesn't mean you are forgetting your circumstances or betraying the person who is gone.

Follow the three e's:

- Exercise. It lifts your mood.
- Eat right. Your body needs fuel even if you never feel hungry anymore.

- Express yourself. Talk about your emotions and feelings if you can. If you can't, try writing in a journal or talking to yourself while having a good cry. Don't hesitate to talk to your doctor or a therapist.

Join a support group. Sometimes you may feel that your grief is a burden to your family or friends. In a support group, you can speak freely with people who are experiencing similar losses.

Do good in someone else's name. Sometimes taking action as a tribute to a loved one helps a lot. Run a race for cancer, donate books to a library in your loved one's name, or plant a special rosebush in your garden. Tributes have a way of bringing some relief to the pain of grief.

We are not suggesting that you measure the course of your feelings against an artificial schedule, but if time has passed—say, four or five months—and you still feel deep, intense grief or depression, or if you're feeling suicidal at any time, it's probably time to talk to someone, perhaps your doctor or social worker or a good friend, about getting professional help to work through your feelings.

Chapter 8

The Health-Care System

Peple who have bladder cancer may have different types of the disease or be in different stages, but they all have one thing in common: before long, they are buried under a blizzard of paperwork and appointments and things to handle.

There are insurance forms. Applications to participate in clinical trials. Prescription refills. Explanations of benefits from the hospital and insurance companies. Instructions on how to prepare for tests or take medications. Forms at work requesting family leave. Maybe you live a fair distance from the hospital and have to arrange for accommodations when you have appointments, or perhaps you need help with child care.

It's overwhelming, and it comes at a time when you may be feeling least able to deal with such demanding issues.

What do you do? Where do you turn for help?

In most cases, your hospital's social work department is a good place to start. You can ask your doctors or nurses for a referral, or you can call the department directly.

At Cleveland Clinic, for example, social workers at the Taussig Cancer Institute can help you sort through many of the topics we'll discuss in this chapter. They can be a lifeline on days when you don't know where to turn. You can reach the Taussig Cancer Institute's social workers through the toll-free Cancer Hotline (866-223-8100).

Insurance and Money Matters

The bills and explanations of benefits and notification of payments from insurance companies or Medicare pile up fast when you are undergoing complex cancer treatment, and it's often difficult to figure out what has been paid, what hasn't, and how much you owe to the hospital, doctors, or service providers such as imaging centers.

Sometimes it seems as if the insurance statements are so hard to understand, they might as well be written in Latin. Social workers can help steer you through the paperwork maze, help you find available financial assistance, and sometimes even act as your advocate in the case of a dispute.

Some people don't receive health insurance as an employment benefit and can't afford to buy it on their own. Others may have exceeded their coverage or have only limited insurance that doesn't cover some tests, treatments, medications, or clinical trials. Maybe you aren't eligible for insurance or aren't working for some reason and simply don't have coverage. Even worse, maybe you can't keep working because of your illness.

Where do you turn for help?

Federal and some state laws protect your rights to buy, use, and keep insurance coverage, but these rights differ depending on variables such as where you live and what kind of insurance you have or want.

Depending on your income level, you might be eligible for Medicaid coverage. If you are disabled and collect Social Security, you might be eligible for a Medicare hospitalization plan, regardless of your age.

If you had to leave your job, you might be able to obtain extended benefits through a state plan called COBRA, which lets you pay to maintain your previous insurance coverage for 18 months after leaving your employer. The U.S. Department of Labor's website at www. dol.gov/ebsa offers information about employer/employee health insurance protections and rights.

There are resources available in certain circumstances for people who have been turned down or have limited (or no) health insurance. A social worker can help you work through the process of finding and applying for these resources, and your state insurance commissioner's office can direct you to state regulations and programs. Check your state's government website and click on the link to the state department of insurance.

You also may be able to apply for an individual health policy during certain periods of the year designated "open enrollment." During these times, you can't be turned down for a preexisting condition. Some insurers or HMOs accept those with preexisting conditions but require a waiting period that can be as long as six months before coverage takes effect.

Ohio has a plan—the Ohio Hospital Care Assurance Program (HCAP)—in place to make sure that people under the federal poverty level who are not enrolled in Medicaid receive free, basic, medically necessary hospital services. Cleveland Clinic goes a step beyond HCAP and gives free hospital services or assistance with financial arrangements for medical care to people without insurance who have income levels up to four times higher than the federal poverty level. In addition, Cleveland Clinic has a financial assistance program that is available to all eligible patients, regardless of whether they have insurance coverage.

Check whether your state government (and the hospital where you are receiving treatment) may have similar assistance plans.

The National Coalition for Cancer Survivorship offers a publication entitled *What Cancer Survivors Need to Know about Health Insurance* that helps patients navigate the financial maze. You can order the publication at the organization's website (www.canceradvocacy.org/resources/publications) or call 877-622-7937 to request a copy. The National Cancer Institute's *Facing Forward: Life after Cancer Treatments* includes a section on insurance issues. It's available at www.cancer.gov, or you can order it by calling 800-422-6237 (800-4-CANCER).

There are additional resources regarding insurance or financial assistance in appendix B of this book.

Got Questions? Get Answers!

The cost of a single day's dose of one of your medications is more than the price of a week's worth of groceries, and you are not sure you can keep taking it because of the expense. Where do you turn? To your doctor? A nurse? A social worker?

If your questions are of a medical nature, talk to your doctor, physician's assistant, or nurse. If you have family concerns, need emotional or financial resources, or want some guidance about how to talk to your loved ones about your cancer, you can also contact your social worker.

The key to getting answers is *asking questions.* You may feel as if your concerns are insignificant or that there is no easy solution. Or perhaps you don't want to bother your doctor or social worker. Don't feel that way. There are amazing resources out there, but if the members of your team don't know about your concern, such as the cost of your daily medication, they can't help you tap into those resources. They want to help you. Doctors, nurses, and social workers all want you to be actively involved in your treatment. Communication between you and your team is paramount.

Communication is more than just asking questions. Getting answers that you understand is equally important. If the answer you receive from your treatment team—whether a response to a medical question or a question about insurance coverage—isn't clear, ask for clarification.

Prepare for conversations or appointments by writing down your questions or concerns and taking notes on the answers. If you want to listen rather than take notes, bring someone (or a tape recorder) along to act as your recording secretary.

Many people feel that they lose control of their lives when they are diagnosed and being treated for cancer. By asking questions and learning about your illness, you can make choices pertaining to your care. Your team can support you in many ways, including by helping you find a support group or information about clinical trials, or guiding you through the maze of insurance coverage or medication assistance.

Financial Assistance for Medications

If you don't have prescription drug insurance coverage, some pharmaceutical companies have programs that make the cost of medications more reasonable. Most companies limit the amount of income you can earn and still be eligible for medication assistance, but the income ceilings are usually much higher than the federal poverty level or the upper limit of Medicaid eligibility.

Don't hesitate to inquire about whether the cost of your prescriptions might be covered through an assistance program, especially if you are doing without food or necessities to buy needed medication—or doing without the medication.

Besides medication assistance for people without a prescription insurance plan and who meet income eligibility requirements, there are low-cost prescription plans provided through many of the pharmaceutical companies for senior citizens enrolled in Medicare and people with disabilities who receive Medicare. Your physician or social worker will be able to advise you about which companies provide such benefits.

Prescription assistance programs work in a variety of ways. In some cases, necessary medications are provided directly through the drug company for either a small fee or sometimes no cost. More often, you are issued a card such as the Orange Card or the Together Rx card, which provides discounts on prescriptions or even some services such as dental and vision.

There are dozens of programs with varying criteria that offer hundreds of covered medications. While that is a good thing for you if you need prescription assistance, it can be confusing to compare the programs and sort out what is covered and how much it will cost you. Luckily, your social worker can help you find sources of medication assistance and is able to help you decide what program best suits your needs.

Searching for Affordable Medications: A Starting Point

If you want to do some research on your own, you can check out eligibility criteria and covered medications by calling a number of organizations toll-free or visiting their websites. Among them are:

- **Needy Meds.** This group lists most major drugs and drug company programs. Applications are available on the website (www.needymeds.com).

(continued on next page)

- **RxAssist.** Similar information is available from this organization, which also offers a comparative chart of most drug-discount programs. (Log on to www. rxassist.org or call 877-844-8442.)

- **Partners for Prescription Assistance (PPARx.org).** This site is a portal to many public and private programs (including programs offered by pharmaceutical companies) that help eligible patients obtain free or nearly free medications. (Log on to www.pparx.org/ Intro.php or call the toll-free number: 888-477-2669 or 888-4PPA-NOW.)

There also are programs sponsored by individual pharmaceutical companies or by consortiums of pharmaceutical companies. Following is a sample listing of available programs:

- **LillyMedicareAnswers** is sponsored by Eli Lilly and Company for patients needing medications not covered by Medicare Part D. Applications are available at the website (www.LillyMedicareAnswers.com) or calling 877-795-4559 or 877-RX-LILLY.

- **Pfizer Sharecard** (www.pfizer.com) is for people age 65 or older or other Medicare enrollees; prescriptions cost a flat fee for a 30-day supply with a Sharecard.

- **SaveWell,** administered by Medical Mutual of Ohio, offers discounted prescriptions as well as discounted vision and dental care. (Log on to www.savewell.com or call 877-728-3935 or 877-SAVEWELL.)

- **Together Rx Card** is open to people on Medicare. The program offers discounted prescriptions from seven major pharmaceutical companies. (Log on to www. togetherrxaccess.com or call 800-444-4106.)

- **Orange Card** is provided through GlaxoSmithKline pharmaceuticals to offer discounts on GSK medications to people on Medicare. Applications can be obtained from health-care providers or by calling 888-672-6436 or 888-ORANGE6.

Patient Support and Advocacy

It is all too easy to feel insignificant when faced with insurance companies, hospital departments, and government agencies. Sometimes, despite everyone's best efforts, you might feel that you aren't getting the treatment or attention you deserve.

How do you voice your concerns and worries when it seems as if everyone else is more important or has more clout than you have?

The first step is to talk to your social worker, who can act as your advocate. That sounds good, but what does "act as your advocate" mean?

The word *advocate* means someone who speaks or acts on your behalf. Someone who takes up your cause and your issues, and who fights for your interests. It means that someone who knows how to get around in the health-care system serves as your voice.

Perhaps your concern is that you feel you need someone to talk to. That you feel alone and adrift and afraid of what is going to happen to you. Your social worker can help you. That's why many hospitals, including Cleveland Clinic, include social work offices in their cancer centers. Social workers are the first to be called in an emotional crisis, and they are able to provide immediate counseling as well as help you find resources such as support groups.

If the idea of telling your feelings and problems to a group doesn't appeal to you, some hospitals have something similar to Cleveland Clinic's 4th Angel program, which pairs bladder-cancer patients (or caregivers) with someone of similar age and sex who has gone through bladder-cancer treatment. The two of you can talk privately and confidentially about what it is like to go through treatment and live with cancer.

Perhaps you are concerned about whether you should participate in a clinical trial. Or perhaps you feel that your case has been mishandled.

While social workers do not make decisions for you or steer you toward making a particular choice, they can and will provide you with all the information you want and need, or they can put you in touch with the appropriate office or individual to answer a question or solve a problem.

Most hospitals, including Cleveland Clinic, have a patient-care center or office of patient support services, where staff members review your medical concerns and talk with doctors, nurses, social workers, or others to resolve your questions and make sure that you are receiving timely and appropriate care.

Most hospitals also have an ombudsman available. An ombudsman is a member of the hospital staff (often trained as a social worker or a nurse) who is available to help you to deal with hospital-based problems or complaints. For example, if you receive a bill for a service you didn't receive, or if you feel that your medical or nursing team is not responding to your concerns or issues appropriately, you can speak confidentially with the ombudsman. After gathering the necessary information, the ombudsman can advise you about the steps to take and sometimes will simply represent your interests to resolve the problem.

There are also public or government organizations that provide advocacy for patient safety:

- If you have a complaint about your doctor, the American Medical Association will investigate and, if appropriate, take action. Contact your state medical board for more information; www.ama-assn.org/ama/pub/category/2645.html provides state links.

- If your concern is about your hospital, surgical center, or laboratory, contact the Joint Commission on Accreditation of Health Care Organizations (http://jcwebnoc.jcaho.org/QMS Internet/IncidentEntry.aspx).

- The U.S. government operates the Agency for Healthcare Research and Quality (www.ahrq.gov), which investigates cases involving patient safety and advocacy.

- The U.S. government's Food and Drug Administration investigates problems with medications or medical devices through its MedWatch reporting system. Their website (www.access data.fda.gov/scripts/medwatch/medwatch-online.htm) provides an online reporting form.

- Some of these agencies may require that you document your complaint or problem with copies of your medical records and supporting information. Federal law gives you the right to obtain a copy of your medical records. For a list of state guides to obtaining medical records, log on to http://medicalrecordrights.georgetown.edu/records.html at the website of Georgetown University's Health Policy Institute.

- The National Institute of Health's Library of Medicine (www.nlm.nih.gov/medlineplus/patient safety. html) offers many additional sources of information about patient safety and advocacy.

Chapter 9

The Future

The future of bladder-cancer diagnosis and management is in the hands of patients and the medical profession.

Perhaps the biggest impediment to progress is the small proportion of patients who enter clinical trials. There are many reasons for this—doctors often are too busy to keep up-to-date with the available trials, and sometimes doctors just don't have connections that allow them to participate directly in clinical trials and they are reluctant to lose contact with their patients. Sometimes patients are fearful or just don't wish to make the commitment. The problem is that progress really only comes through clinical investigation, and at present not even 10 percent of eligible patients participate in the available studies.

Most promising for the future is the development of some of the novel targeted therapies, those that have been developed based upon our understanding of the biology of cancer, particularly the biochemistry and genetics of cancer. As mentioned previously, agents that are targeted on the inhibition of genes that control cancer growth (such as the epidermal growth factor receptor) and enzymes responsible for angiogenesis and cancer growth (such as the tyrosine kinase inhibitors) are perhaps the most promising current strategies.

We know that immunological stimulation, such as that offered by BCG for superficial bladder cancer, has been helpful in causing shrinkage of bladder cancer. There are a number of proteins that have been identified in the bladder that might constitute targets for immunological therapy, and clinical trials testing some of these new reagents are in progress.

In addition, several classes of novel anticancer compounds within the category of cytotoxic chemotherapy have recently been identified and as of this writing and are in phase I and phase II testing, trying to identify the safe dosage and likely anticancer effects against bladder cancer.

Another important area in the development of future strategies of cancer care will be in the area of molecular diagnostics. This involves the development of pathology tests that can identify specific genes or molecules within cancer cells that indicate prognosis or potential response to specific therapies.

For example, preliminary studies suggested that the P53 gene, a gene that suppresses cancer growth, can sometimes be mutated (or altered) in cancer of the bladder. Studies at the University of Southern California suggested that mutation of the P53 gene can be identified by a pathological test, that cancers with such mutations have a worse prognosis, and paradoxically that cancers with some of these mutations can actually have a better response to chemotherapy than those without the mutations. This set of observations was the subject of a large randomized trial that studied P53 mutations and response to chemotherapy in bladder cancer. That trial recently closed. The publication of these results may be important in shaping design strategies for future bladder-cancer trials.

What is very apparent is that our understanding of the drivers of cancer has become much clearer with our improved knowledge of the human genome (the components of the genes within the human body). As we design better drugs that are focused on the mechanisms of cancer growth, clinical trials will offer a greater potential for cure. However, this potential will also require our community, including patients, their families, and their doctors, to support the available trials, leading to a time when advanced bladder cancer is no longer such a threat.

Acknowledgments

The authors would like to thank Cleveland Clinic and the Cleveland Clinic Press staff for providing information, resources, and support. Our thanks go as well to Jennifer Stonebrook of the Hospice of the Western Reserve and to Judy Levendula, L.I.S.W., and the hospice team of Cleveland Clinic for their generous interviews.

Special thanks to Mary Jo Gurin of Cleveland Clinic
for her generous help in getting this
manuscript "to the end."
—KT

Appendix A

What Is Cancer?

Cancer is not one disease; it is many diseases affecting parts of the human body. All cancers have one thing in common: something has gone wrong in the way some of the body's cells normally grow, divide, and die.

In a healthy body, normal cells divide as new cells are needed (*mitosis*) and self-destruct when the cells become old or damaged (*apoptosis*).

Sometimes, however, exposure to chemicals (e.g., cigarette smoke), radiation, sunlight, or even rare types of virus infections, as well as heredity, can damage our DNA, those building blocks of our bodies that store our genetic material (genes).

When DNA is damaged, the genes that control cell growth may malfunction. Cells that normally act as stoplights during cell growth and division may break down. Sometimes the damage leads to the development of *oncogenes*, which stimulate uncontrolled cell growth. Sometimes the DNA damage leads to the absence of genes called *suppressor* genes, which normally function by preventing abnormal cells from growing into tumors.

When DNA is damaged and uncontrolled growth occurs, cancer cells invade the body. Sometimes the cancer cells cluster together to form a tumor. Tumors are *solid cancers* that affect the body's organs, such as the lungs, breast, bowel, prostate, or bladder. Sometimes the cancer cells don't form tumors and are *liquid*, circulating in the bloodstream to cause cancers of the lymphatic and blood systems.

Cancers may remain clustered in a tumor or a specific area of the body, or they may invade surrounding or distant parts of the body.

In order to grow, tumors must build a system of blood vessels, a process called *angiogenesis.* Sometimes this process is interrupted by a physical, pharmaceutical, or chemical cause, and the tumor remains dormant.

Other times, the cancer cells or tumor do grow and may even invade other parts of the body. Sometimes cancer cells from an established tumor spread to surrounding tissue (*invasion*) or are transported through the bloodstream to other areas of the body (*metastasis*). Bladder-cancer cells may metastasize to the liver, for example, and tumors may appear there, although the tumors will still be bladder-cancer cells even though they are physically located in the liver.

Different types of cancer behave differently. Even within a particular cancer type, such as bladder cancer, different forms of the disease have different characteristics and respond differently to treatment.

Appendix B

Websites and Resources

While every effort has been made to suggest websites that are up-to-date, accurate, and professional, we recommend that you evaluate the sites to determine your level of confidence in the data provided. As recommended elsewhere in this book, discuss *any* websites with your doctor before relying on the information provided on the website.

Evaluating Websites

Cancer Index also provides a short evaluation form (at www.cancerindex.org/clinks18.htm) to help you determine whether websites are trustworthy and up-to-date.

The National Library of Medicine funds www.eaccesshealth.org/training/issues.html, a website that discusses how to determine if you should trust medical information published on a website. It includes a section on sites that are *not* recommended and links to services such as Quackwatch.

Advanced Directives

FindLaw
http://estate.findlaw.com/estate-planning/living-wills.html
Information on living wills.

National Hospice and Palliative Care Organization
www.nhpco.org
800-658-8898
Links to state-by-state advanced directives, hospice programs, and Caring Connections, a comprehensive section on end-of-life issues.

Ohio Hospice and Palliative Care Organization
http://ohpco.org
800-776-9513
Links to hospices by city/area, with resources for hospice professionals as well as for families and hospice patients.

General Sites

The sites in this section include information about cancer. Many of these sites offer specific links to or information about bladder cancer, and some include extensive information not only on cancer, but also on support groups, grief, nutrition, oncology drugs, and clinical trials as well. Please discuss these sites and information you obtain from them with your doctor.

American Cancer Society
www.cancer.org
800-227-2345 or 800-ACS-2345
Includes the Cancer Survivors Network, a forum/message board where you can ask questions, share information and resources, and talk with other people who are dealing with cancer.

American Medical Association
www.ama-assn.org
800-621-8335
Includes a Doctor Finder and information on medical ethics.

American Society of Clinical Oncology
www.asco.org
A professional medical website that includes a section titled *PLWC, People Living with Cancer* (www.plwc.org/portal/site/PLWC).

Bladder Cancer Web Café
http://blcwebcafe.org/default.aspi
Inspiring stories of bladder-cancer survivors as well as online forums, resources, and information on bladder cancer.

CancerCare
www.cancercare.org
800-813-4673 or 800-813-HOPE
A nonprofit organization offering free professional support, including online support groups, for people with cancer.

Cancer Help Online
www.cancerhelponline.org
Links to extensive cancer resources.

Cancer Index
www.cancerindex.org
A list of online cancer resources maintained by volunteers; the specific index for bladder cancer maintained on this site can be found at www.cancerindex.org/clinks3d.htm.

Chemocare.com
www.chemocare.com
Packed with information on how to manage chemotherapy and side effects as well as how to bank sperm, what to expect from various chemotherapy regimens, and much more. This website is affiliated with the program established by cancer survivor and Olympic gold medalist Scott Hamilton, the Scott Hamilton CARES Initiative, which can be found at www.clevelandclinic.org/cancer/scottcares.

Hospice of the Western Reserve
www.hospicewr.org
800-707-8922
Resources for caregivers, patients, and professionals.

Medline Plus
www.nlm.nih.gov/medlineplus
Detailed resources on cancer from the National Institutes of Health; includes a link to help you find local resources in your area.

National Cancer Institute
www.cancer.gov
800-422-6237 or 800-4-CANCER
Extensive resources include downloadable brochures, newsletters, a drug information list, live online help, and help finding a doctor for a second opinion.

National Coalition for Cancer Survivorship
www.canceradvocacy.org
877-622-7937 or 877-NCCS-YES
Includes an audio section entitled "The Cancer Survival Toolbox."

National Institutes of Health
www.nih.gov
301-496-4000
Comprehensive website with resources on a wide range of cancer topics, information on clinical trials, and hotlines.

National Women's Health Information Center
www.4women.gov
800-994-9662
General health information for women and girls from the U.S. Department of Health and Human Services.

Office of Minority Health
www.omhrc.gov
800-444-6472
Resources and information for African Americans, Native Americans, Latinos, Asian Americans, Hawaiians/Pacific Islanders.

Ohio Hospice and Palliative Care Organization
http://ohpco.org
800-776-9513
Links to hospices by city/area, with resources for hospice professionals as well as for families and hospice patients.

The Wellness Community
www.thewellnesscommunity.org
888-793-9355 or 888-793-WELL
Extensive resources, information about clinical trials, online support groups, and webcasts.

Second Opinions

The American Board of Medical Specialties
www.abms.org
Lists certified doctors on its website. (Click on the section for consumers.)

Cleveland Clinic
www.clevelandclinic.org/quality/choose/second.htm
800-223-2273
Offers an article discussing when and how to get a second opinion.

National Cancer Institute
www.cancer.gov/cancertopics/wyntk/ bladder/page9
800-422-6237 or 800-4-CANCER
Includes a referral service to treatment centers it supports.
Also includes an article on getting a second opinion when the diagnosis is specifically bladder cancer.

Clinical Trials

Besides **Cleveland Clinic,** www.clevelandclinic.org/cancer, and the links provided in chapter 6, the following websites have information on clinical trials, whether to participate, how to find and evaluate programs, and what's new:

American Association for Cancer Research
www.aacr.org
A cancer dictionary, information on clinical trials, and the latest research.

National Cancer Institute
www.cancer.gov
800-422-6237 or 800-4-CANCER

U.S. National Institutes of Health and the **National Library of Medicine**
ww.clinicaltrials.gov
Information on federally funded and privately funded clinical trials, searchable by disease, sponsor, and recruitment status.

Coping with Cancer and Grief

American Cancer Society
www.cancer.org
800-227-2345 or 800-ACS-2345
Information on coping with cancer, from diagnosis and treatment issues to managing everyday life; includes the Cancer Survivors Network, videos, and personal stories about coping with cancer.

Books for children about cancer
www.cancer.med.umich.edu/learn/pwtalking.htm
A reading list provided by the University of Michigan.

CancerCare
www.cancercare.org
800-813-4673
Features a "reading room" with articles for people with cancer, loved ones, and caregivers; online support groups; and a Get Help section with online support.

Caregivers Library
www.caregiverslibrary.org
Articles, lists, and resources on caregiving, end-of-life issues, and emotional support.

Cleveland Clinic 4th Angel Program
www.clevelandclinic.org/cancer/scottcares/4thangel/about.asp
800-223-2273, ext. 52573

Offers a nationwide mentorship program for those with cancer and their caregivers; part of the Scott Hamilton CARES Initiative at Cleveland Clinic.

Cleveland Clinic Social Work Department
www.clevelandclinic.org/socialwork
216-444-6552

Cleveland Clinic Taussig Cancer Institute
http://my.clevelandclinic.org/cancer/default.aspx
866-223-8100 (Cancer Answer Line)
Comprehensive cancer information and resources.

Crisis, Grief & Healing
http://webhealing.com
Online discussion boards for people dealing with grief and healing, excerpts of books and columns on grief, particularly for men, by a nationally recognized psychotherapist.

Gillette Cancer Connection
www.gillettecancerconnect.org
Sections for men and for women on living with cancer; offers downloadable brochures, including *When Someone You Love Has Cancer: A Guide for Families.*

Growth House
http://growthhouse.org
A resource on end of life and death with dignity; offers an online bookstore with topical titles and Quiet Music, a restful online radio channel.

Intimate Moments
www.intimatemomentsapparel.com.
Intimate and sports apparel for people with urinary pouches.

Look Good, Feel Better
http://lookgoodfeelbetter.org
800-395-5665 (800-395-LOOK)
Practical guides on personal appearance for men, women, and teens with cancer are available at the website or through a mail

order video. Look Good, Feel Better also hosts local live programs, where participants can interact face-to-face throughout the world; the website includes a program locator.

Mayo Clinic
www.mayoclinic.com/health/cancer-treatment/SA00071
Addresses the sexual side effects of cancer for women.
www.mayoclinic.com/health/cancer-treatment/SA00070
Addresses the sexual side effects of cancer for men.

National Cancer Institute
www.cancer.gov/cancertopics/coping
800-422-6237 or 800-4-CANCER
Addresses comprehensive topics such as side effects, emotional concerns, pain, nutrition, and end-of-life concerns; includes an article on talking with children and teens about cancer: www.cancer.gov/cancertopics/When-Someone-You-Love-Is-Treated/page6.

National Coalition for Cancer Survivorship
www.canceradvocacy.org
877-622-7937
Includes an audio section entitled "The Cancer Survival Toolbox."

National Family Caregivers Association
www.nfcacares.org
Tips, guides, and articles for caregivers.

National Hospice and Palliative Care Organization
www.nhpco.org
800-658-8898
Links to state-by-state advance directives and hospice programs, and features Caring Connections, a comprehensive section on end of life.

OncoLink
www.oncolink.com/coping/index.cfm
Comprehensive information about cancer for patients, caregivers, and loved ones; includes an online ask-the-expert section and a section for newly diagnosed patients.

Wound Ostomy and Continence Nurses Society

ww.wocn.org
888-224-9626
Links to many apparel companies that design for people with urinary pouches are available on the website.

Drug Assistance and Oncology Drugs

Federal Food and Drug Administration
www.fda.gov/cder/cancer/index.htm
Oncology drug research and evaluation website, including a list of approved oncology drugs.

Needy Meds
www.needymeds.com
Lists most major drugs and drug company programs.

RxAssist
www.rxassist.org
877-844-8442
Lists drugs and drug company programs, with a chart comparing most drug-discount programs.

Partners for Prescription Assistance
https://www.pparx.org/Intro.php
888-477-2669 or 888-4PPA-NOW
An interactive website sponsored by the Pharmaceutical Research and Manufacturers of America (PhRMA, www.phrma.org); links to hundreds of public and private programs helping eligible patients obtain free or nearly free medications.

There are also programs sponsored by individual pharmaceutical companies or by consortiums of pharmaceutical companies. This is a sample listing of some of the available programs:

LillyMedicareAnswers
www.LillyMedicareAnswers.com
877-795-4559 or 877-RX-LILLY
Sponsored by Eli Lilly and Company for patients needing medications not covered by Medicare Part D.

Pfizer Sharecard

www.pfizer.com

For people age 65 or older or other Medicare enrollees.

SaveWell

www.savewell.com

877-728-3935 or 877-SAVEWELL

Administered by Medical Mutual of Ohio; offers discounted prescriptions as well as discounted vision and dental care.

Together Rx Card

www.togetherrxaccess.com

800-444-4106

Open to seniors and other people on Medicare; offers discounted prescriptions from seven major pharmaceutical companies.

Orange Card

www.orangecard.com

888-672-6436 or 888-ORANGE6

Offers assistance for seniors and people on Medicare through GlaxoSmithKline pharmaceuticals.

Government Agencies

Centers for Disease Control

www.cdc.gov/cancer

Cancer statistics and resources for cancer prevention and control.

Medicaid

www.cms.hhs.gov/home/medicaid.asp

Comprehensive links to information about Medicaid health care.

Medicare

www.medicare.gov

800-633-4227

Medicare Rights Center

www.medicarerights.org
An independent nonprofit consumer source of health-care information counseling, including a hotline for Medicare questions and an enrollment program for people who need help with medical care costs.

Social Security Administration

www.ssa.gov
800-772-1213
Information on Medicare, the Medicare prescription drug plan, disability insurance, and Supplemental Security Income (SSI).

U.S. Department of Health and Human Services

www.dhhs.gov
877-696-6775
Resources on drugs, bioethics, clinical trials, coping and support, alternative medicine, and specific diseases.

Help with Insurance, Financial Assistance, or Employment

Association of Community Cancer Centers

www.accc-cancer.org
301-984-9496
Offers article "Cancer Treatments Your Insurance Should Cover."

CancerCare

www.cancercare.org/get_help/assistance/index.php
800-813-4673
Includes a printable booklet, *A Helping Hand*, which includes resources and tips for finding financial assistance.

Civil Rights Offices

http://public.findlaw.com/civil-rights/civil-rights-resources/state-civil-rights-offices.html
A list of state civil rights offices that can respond to discrimination complaints.

Healthinsuranceinfo.net
www.healthinsuranceinfo.net
A nonprofit website dedicated to how to get and keep health insurance; includes guides to managing medical bills and state-by-state consumer health guides written by the Georgetown University Health Policy Institute.

National Association of Insurance Commissioners
www.naic.org
816-842-3600
Information about state insurance offices and links to state departments of insurance.

National Coalition for Cancer Survivorship
www.canceradvocacy.org/resources/publications
301-650-8868
Includes the article "What Cancer Survivors Need to Know about Health Insurance."

Patient Advocate Foundation
www.patientadvocate.org
800-532-5274
A national nonprofit organization helping patients deal with insurance companies, manage debt crisis, and liaise with employers; online support.

State Health Insurance Assistance Programs
www.shiptalk.org
A counseling program with information about health-insurance assistance for Medicare recipients.

U.S. Department of Labor
www.dol.gov
866-487-2365 or 866-4-USA-DOL
Information on Family Leave Act, COBRA insurance, Americans with Disabilities Act, and the Rehabilitation Act.

Miscellaneous Resources

Air Charity Network

http://aircharitynetwork.org

Executive offices: 877-858-7788; to request assistance: 877-621-7177

Assistance to people in need of free air transportation to specialized health-care facilities.

Cancer Patient Travel

www.cancerpatienttravel.org

Travel/administrative office: 757-318-9174; travel/patient phone: 800-296-1217; lodging: 800-542-9730

Charitable long-distance travel and lodging for cancer patients in need.

Hope Lodge

www.cancer.org/docroot/SHR/content/SHR_2.1_x_Hope_Lodge.asp

Provided by the American Cancer Society; helps with housing for families who need to be away from home for cancer treatment.

Joe's House

www.joeshouse.org

877-563-7468

A nonprofit organization specializing in accommodations for traveling cancer patients.

Online Medical and Health Information

AARP

www.aarp.org/health/staying_healthy/prevention/a2003-03-17-wwwhealth.html

Offers an article "Finding Health Information Online."

Health on the Net Foundation

www.hon.ch/HONcode/HONcode_check.html

Provides the "Code of Conduct for Medical and Health Websites."

The Medical Library Association
http://mlanet.org/resources/medspeak/topten.html
A list of its top ten most useful medical websites.

National Library of Medicine
Funds the website www.eaccesshealth.org/training/issues.html.

Quackwatch
www.quackwatch.org
A nonprofit website.

Appendix C

Using Medical Information from the Internet

B efore you take information you have read on the Internet as fact, make sure the websites you visit are reputable and that the site is current and updated. Some doctors maintain lists of reputable websites and give the information to patients who are interested in researching their diagnosis or treatment. In all cases, discuss any information you find online or elsewhere with your doctor.

Some things to look for when surfing the Web for medical information:

- **Accuracy:** Can you verify the information elsewhere? Are sources cited? Are the sources professional?

- **Authority:** Who is the author? What are the author's credentials?

- **Objectivity:** Are there indications that the site wants to sell you something? Does it appear to have an agenda of some sort?

- **Timeliness:** When was the website last updated? Is it current? Are articles dated?

- **Principles:** Does the website state that it does not take the place of a doctor/patient relationship? Does it disclose any conflict of interest? Is advertising clearly marked as such? Is the website source a non-profit group, a government agency, or a professional health organization? Is there a clearly identified way of contacting the webmaster or professionals cited on the website? Does it ask for any personal information, and if so, how does it protect confidential information?

Use the information you find to prepare questions for your medical team, educate yourself about a particular disease, and investigate helpful resources for such issues as insurance questions, finding a doctor or medical facility, and researching clinical trials. Do not use the information you find to diagnose yourself or self-prescribe a treatment plan. Websites are resources meant to enhance, not replace, health-care professionals.

Discuss the websites you visit and information you find with your doctor, but don't debate it or challenge his expertise. If your doctor feels that you are trying to put him or her on the spot rather than discuss your concerns or ask questions about information that you don't understand, he or she may become defensive. For example, don't bring 50 or 60 pages of research to your next appointment and expect your doctor to read them. If you find an article from a reputable site that you want to discuss with your doctor, bring the relevant citation only, along with confirmation of the author and website's authenticity.

As an indication of the extent of the information available on the Internet, and the desire by providers that patients take the time to inform themselves, many hospitals and large medical practices make computers available for patients to use on-site.

You deserve a physician who values an educated, empowered patient, yet you don't want to empower yourself to the point of being an antagonist. It's a delicate balancing act for both patients and doctors, because while the Internet can be an important tool in the doctor/patient relationship, it can also be a wedge in the communication process and can, if not used properly, interfere with your getting the best information available about your disease, diagnosis, and treatment.

Here are some websites devoted to the safe use of the Internet for medical research:

www.eaccesshealth.org/training/issues.html
A website funded by the National Library of Medicine.

http://mlanet.org/resources/medspeak/topten.html
The Medical Library Association's list of its top ten medical websites.

www.quackwatch.org
Quackwatch, a nonprofit website.

www.aarp.org/health/staying_healthy/prevention/a2003-03-17-wwwhealth.html
"Finding Health Information Online," an article on the AARP website.

www.hon.ch/HONcode/HONcode_check.html
The Code of Conduct for Medical and Health Websites provided by Health on the Net Foundation.

Here are some websites that both physicians and patients might find useful:

www.medstory.com
A search engine for medical information.

www.merckhomeedition.com
Site of the *Merck Manual of Medical Information.*

www.medem.com
An interactive site founded by the American Medical Association.

Appendix D

How to Talk to Your Doctor

Throughout this book we have talked about the importance of communicating with your doctor and discussing your questions and concerns during your journey through bladder cancer.

But engaging with your doctor might not seem like such a simple process to you. Perhaps you have been referred to a new doctor, a urologist, who is recommending chemotherapy and surgery. You may wonder whether he or she even knows your name, and sometimes you feel as if the doctor is rushing you because the next appointment is already waiting in the room down the hall. Yet this doctor holds your life in his or her hands.

You would like to communicate. But how?

Preparing for your doctor visits, especially during the diagnostic phase when you may be seeing a new doctor or a new team of doctors, is a good first step on your part. One way to prepare is to organize your medical information. Buy a three-ring notebook with some dividers in it, lots of blank sheets of notebook paper, and a three-hole paper punch. Mark the dividers with categories such as Medication, Tests and Results, Office Visits, Questions, Contacts. You'll devise more categories as time goes by.

Take the notebook with you to appointments and even treatments if you want. Keep track of doctors' names, when you underwent tests, and when you started and stopped a particular treatment. Tape business cards or appointment reminders into the notebook, too. You'll have everything in one place, and it will help not only you but sometimes your doctor to keep track of things.

Keep track of your questions in your notebook; leave space to jot down a short answer. Some people use tape recorders to record their doctors' answers to questions. (Ask your doctor if he or she minds; most don't.) Other patients prefer to bring someone with them to act as extra ears. In either case, transfer the information you receive during your appointment to your notebook.

Be sure to ask your doctor to write down or spell unfamiliar medical terms. Having the correct spelling at hand will allow you to look up new terms in a medical dictionary. (A good online dictionary can be found at www.nlm.nih. gov/medlineplus/mplusdictionary.html.)

Ask your questions in simple terms: What is wrong with me? What do I do if this treatment fails? What does that drug do? Do I need a follow-up visit? If you put your question in simple terms, you are more likely to receive an answer that is also couched in simple terms.

Sometimes doctors are so stressed by the pressures of their own lives, whether business or professional, that they hurry or become impatient. It's only human, but if you don't understand something, ask the doctor to repeat the information. If you feel intimidated, remember: this is your life, your cancer, and you need to get answers. You *deserve* to have answers. Politely ask for an explanation.

And do be truthful. If you have four beers every night, don't fudge and say two. Smoking three cigarettes a week is still smoking, and a herbal supplement that you take to help you sleep can interact with other drugs; be sure you mention these things.

Don't hesitate to call the doctor's office if you forget to ask something or have a problem. If you want to talk to the doctor, not a nurse, it's reasonable to be firm, leave your number, and ask to be called back. It's not reasonable to demand that the doctor come to the phone while you wait.

Whether you are a new patient building a relationship with a new doctor or you are seeing the same doctor you've been going to for years, communication takes respect and a willingness to be open and professional.

It's well worth it.

Bibliography

The following represents a partial list of resources employed in the creation of this book.

Print Resources

Droller, M. J., ed. *American Cancer Society Atlas of Clinical Oncology: Urothelial Tumors.* Hamilton, Out.: B. C. Decker, 2004.

Grossman, H. B., Natale, R. B., Tangen, C. M., et al. SWOG 8710 (INT-0080)—"Randomized phase III trial of neoadjuvant methotrexate, vinblastine, doxorubicin, and cisplatin + cystectomy versus cystectomy alone in patients with locally advanced bladder cancer." *New England Journal of Medicine* 349 (2003): 859–866.

Raghavan, D., and Bailey, M. J. *Bladder Cancer—Fast Facts*, 2nd ed. London: Health Press, 2005.

Raghavan, D., and Huben, R. "Management of bladder cancer." *Current Problems in Cancer* 19 (1995):1–64.

Raghavan, D., Scher, H., Leibel, S., and Lange. P. *Principles and Practice of Genitourinary Oncology*. Philadelphia: J. B. Lippincott-Raven, 1997.

Resnick. M., and Novick, A. *Urology Secrets*, 3rd ed. Philadelphia: Hanley & Belfus, 2002.

Stein, J. P., Lieskovsky, G., Cote, R., et al. "Radical cystectomy in the treatment of invasive bladder cancer: Long-term results in 1,054 patients." *Journal of Clinical Oncology* 19 (2001): 666–675.

Online Resources
American Cancer Society
www.cancer.org
Numerous articles, including (but not limited to) "Managing Your Cancer Experience," "Support Programs and Services," "Learn about Cancer," "Clinical Trials," and "Treatment Decision Tools."

American Society of Clinical Oncology
www.plwc.org
"People Living with Cancer," "Guide to Living with Bladder Cancer," and other articles.

Cleveland Clinic
www.clevelandclinic.org
Materials provided at the website and other materials published by Cleveland Clinic, including the home pages for Bladder Cancer, Clinical Trials, the Glickman Urological and Kidney Institute, the Scott Hamilton CARES Initiative, the sociology department, and the Taussig Cancer Institute.

National Cancer Institute
www.cancer.gov
Numerous articles, including (but not limited to) "Cancer Topics," "Clinical Trials and Insurance Coverage: A Resource

Guide," "Bladder Cancer," "Coping with Cancer," and "Cancer Statistics."

National Hospice and Palliative Care Organization
www.nhpco.org
Numerous articles, including (but not limited to) "Learn about End of Life Care," "Advance Directives," and "Caring Connections."

National Institutes of Health
http://health.nih.gov
Numerous articles, including (but not limited to) Bladder Cancer home page, "What You Need to Know about Bladder Cancer," "General Cancer Resources," and "Dictionary of Cancer Terms."

National Institutes of Health/National Library of Medicine
Clinical trials home page: www.clinicaltrials.gov

Index

Cleveland Clinic

Cleveland Clinic, located in Cleveland, Ohio, is a not-for-profit multispecialty academic medical center that integrates clinical and hospital care with research and education. Cleveland Clinic was founded in 1921 by four renowned physicians with a vision of providing outstanding patient care based upon the principles of cooperation, compassion, and innovation. *U.S. News & World Report* consistently names Cleveland Clinic as one of the nation's best hospitals in its annual America's Best Hospitals survey. The Glickman Urological & Kidney Institute is a world leader in treating complex urologic and kidney conditions in adults and children and has been ranked as one of the top programs in the nation for urological care by *U.S. News & World Report* every year since 2000. Approximately 1,800 full-time salaried physicians and scientists at Cleveland Clinic and Cleveland Clinic Florida represent more than 120 medical specialties and subspecialties. Every year, patients come for treatment from every state and more than 80 countries around the world.

www.clevelandclinic.org